The Self-Treatment techniques in this book ... helped thousands of athletes continue their sport and be

Pain Free

The Pain-Free Runner

Julie Donnelly, LMT
and
Zev M. Cohen, MD

Makai Press, Suffern, New York

The Pain-Free Runner

By: Julie Donnelly, LMT and Zev M. Cohen, MD

Published by:
Makai Press
15 Wesley Chapel Road
Suffern, NY 10901
www.julstro.com
SAN: 2 5 5 - 4 1 6 X
Senior Editor: Jerry Trump
Book Layout: Textype, Inc.
Photographer: Jerry Trump and Julie Donnelly
Illustrator: Jerry Trump
Library of Congress Control Number: 2003106725
Donnelly, Julie and Cohen, Zev
    The Pain-Free Runner
ISBN: 0-9741969-0-8
    1. Self-Help 2. Education & Teaching 3. Health & Fitness 4. Title

Legal Information

The content of this manual is furnished for informational use only. It is not meant to replace medical care. WARINING: Many injuries and conditions are serious and require medical treatment by a qualified physician. Contact your physician prior to using the Julstro Techniques. Use of the treatments and/or programs in this book are done at the user's discretion.

Dedicated

To

The Pursuit of Health and Wellness

TABLE OF CONTENTS

FOREWORDS

Jerry Trump

Have you ever had this happen to you – you spend years believing in a given "truth," or even doing something the same way for most of your life? Then "it" happens. It may be an event of some kind. Or someone you meet. It happens by accident. And then a whole new reality is upon you. You are faced with the realization that you have been completely blind. Out in the dark. Missing the boat.

So what am I talking about? I have been involved in athletics all my life. I can't remember a time when I wasn't on the Little League field, or doing whatever sport was in season. By the time I had reached college, I had been misfortunate enough to receive more than one "career ending" injury and multiple surgeries.

I still managed to play basketball at a NCAA division 1 level college, spending as much time in the care of sports trainers and doctors, as just about anybody. The point to this is that I've injured just about every part of my body at one time or another, playing one sport or another. Over the years, I've come to know the routine of treating sports related injuries quite well. Some of which I have overcome, and some of which I had come to the conclusion that I would have to live with. Over the last couple of years however, it meant not being able to train enough to compete in an Ironman distance triathlon. A dream that I had concluded would go unfulfilled.

I met Julie Donnelly completely by accident. I had given up on finding someone who could treat my Achilles Tendonitis with results. It would always re-occur with any lengthy training sessions. Julie sent me her book.

And that's when I had "it" happen to me. I found myself following directions and treating the mid-calf area of my leg, not my heel, (where all the pain was coming from). "How could that work?" From the time I had my first "booboo" the question was "where does it hurt?" and then the attention always focused on that area. And most certainly throughout my sports life, I don't remember one doctor fooling with a small spot on a muscle more that a foot away from my injury.

To keep this story short, here is the result. My $300.00 pair of prescription orthotics is in the closet, and I finished my first Ironman Triathlon in June of 2002. This is completely due to Julie's technique of treating repetitive strain injuries.

Julie Donnelly is not only an insightful and knowledgeable therapist, but she is also a teacher in the true sense of the word. I encourage you to take this book and use it as a guide to better health, better performance, and a better life. Don't be shocked to find that the pain in your shoulder just might be caused by a spasm in your back; and that you can treat it in a matter of minutes, not weeks.

Just remember that the recognized experts in the field used to think that the earth was flat.

 Jerry Trump

Paul Watson

If you've ever had an injury that continually resurfaced after seemingly successful rehabilitation, or just one that refused to go away regardless of the various treatments, this book may very well hold the answers to your mysteries.

For nearly a decade I had dedicated hours of my daily schedule to rigorous training in pursuit of world-class physical conditioning necessary for highly competitive swimming, running, and rough-terrain racing events.

Over these years I had my share of strains, pulls, and bruises along the way but felt nearly invincible and confident nothing could keep me down.

However, I began injuring the area around my biceps-tendon on a regular basis, which routinely sidelined me from engaging in any meaningful swim training. Just when it was completely healed and I was confident it was 100%, sometimes for weeks, I would restrain it again. I thus began what turned out to be an exhaustive search of the healthcare industry for help. I saw orthopedists, massage therapists, neurologists, and chiropractors—in addition to having x-rays, MRI's, physical therapy, acupuncture, and ancient Chinese qui-gong performed on it—all to no avail. The "tendonitis" (as it was labeled) returned every time, shortly following the often-lengthy rehabilitation a "specialist" prescribed.

It took Julie Donnelly exactly two emails for her to correctly diagnose and solve this mystery. The problem: a shortening of the biceps muscle. The likely reason: all the aggressive swim training (hard intervals, weighted pull-ups, etc.). The solution: stretching. Hard to believe, isn't it? How could something so simple be so effective? Well, the advice and instruction not only worked for once, but also made perfect sense. The muscle was becoming shortened as a result of being in a prolonged state of contraction (2-4 hour swim workouts, 500 or so pull-ups over 90 minutes, etc.).

Not all of life's stories have a happy ending. Fortunately for me, this one does as I've seen these treatments work on me. If you are experiencing any training-related injuries, chances are great this book will help you successfully cure them. Follow the basic instructions she presents for any area that you have injured or have discomfort.

Finally this book can act as an exceptional preventative tool and I encourage you to read through it and take advantage of her knowledge.

Your training will surely benefit.

Paul Watson
Winner of 1999 "Beast of the East" competition

ACKNOWLEDGMENTS

Julie Donnelly, BS, LMT

This series of Pain-Free books has become a true "Work in Progress"!

It all began in 1993 with some simple notes for my clients, many of whom were athletes and needed to learn how to immediately stop a pain that occurred during a training session, or a competition.

The next step, taken in 1999, was to gather together all the various notes I had written, and publish it as "How To Be Painless...A Beginner's Guide to the Self Treatment of Muscle Spasms". The models in this original book were real clients from my office, people of every age and body type, all of whom received benefit from the treatments. In fact, many of the treatments in the book were developed specifically for them!

In December 2001, Jerry Trump, an Ironman Triathlete with a severe Achilles tendonitis condition, found my book – and that was the beginning of this series. I'm glad to say that Jerry did successfully compete in the 2002 Utah Ironman Competition, and went on to finish a second Ironman event! We wish him Good Luck and Good Health with his continuing athletic efforts.

After Jerry learned how to successfully self-treat the source of his

Achilles Tendonitis, he convinced me to help athletes by going onto various forums, and that work became an eBook, "The Pain-Free Triathlete", and led to separate sport specific volumes. With this format, athletes will be able to focus on the muscles that they use the most. Jerry moved the entire Julstro Self-Treatment System to a new area that is exciting for me – working hand-in-hand with dedicated athletes through books, consultations, and Julstro Self Treatment Clinics both in gyms, and at major sporting events around the USA.

There are many people who have made this series of books become a reality, and I want to thank each person who has been a springboard for growth.

My wonderful family: my children Anne-Marie & Michael, their loving spouses Rob & Colleen, and the light of my life, my grandchildren: Meaghan, Ellen, Jack, Martin, Kate and Aidan. Thank you for listening to me as I endlessly went on & on "creating in my mind". You believed in me and loved me. I really appreciate how you inspired me.

I especially want to acknowledge my late friend, Beth, for teaching me that I was more than I believed. She started me on the road to an education, and was my constant cheering section. I know she sees this from her higher vantage point, and is smiling at me.

Zev Cohen, MD has been my supporter, my friend, and my toughest editor! He realized the value of what I was offering, long before the medical community would entertain the idea that muscles cause joint pain, and other chronic painful conditions. He invited me into his medical office to work with his patients, and showed me the perfect union between medicine and muscle therapy – I appreciate him immensely. The relationship has opened doors that I could only dream about – and we have both changed because of our mutual respect for each other.

His full participation in the self-treatment of Carpal Tunnel Syndrome was the catalyst to bringing this vital information out of the office, and into the homes of people around the world. We have proven that the pain and numbness associated with Carpal Tunnel Syndrome can be eliminated after just a few self-treatments! We have truly made a difference in the way this condition is being treated medically. We will continue our efforts until Carpal Tunnel Syndrome is no longer thought of as a debilitating condition.

Jerry Trump has been the catalyst for this stage in my growth - aside from inspiring me to write these books, Jerry's artistic ability is responsible for the beautiful graphics, and muscle drawings, that are used throughout all of the books, and for making the word "Julstro" become synonymous with relief from muscle &/or joint pain.

There were several others who have made this work become a reality. Special thanks go to:

*   Paul Froehlich – for being one of the first people to believe in the Julstro Techniques, and for all the direction and hard work you did to support and inspire me. Thanks for helping to put "Julstro" into a video format, and into homes everywhere.

*   Shawn Boom – we appreciate his excellent chapters on exercises specific to each book title.

*   JoAnn Dahlkoetter, Ph.D. – For her chapter on paying attention to your body; often overlooked, but extremely important.

*   Sue Kopac – for keeping the office running; finding lost objects, understanding my "multiple #1 priorities" and making sense out of them; doing her best to make the computer "user friendly"; and finally, for listening to me as I go into my excited visionary world!

*   Our models: Paul Watson, Greg Smith, Megan Bussart, Jerry Trump, Becky Thurn, and Bernie Casserly - all athletes who use the Julstro System on a daily basis, and have made the descriptions come alive. We appreciate their support!

Finally, speaking for both Dr. Cohen and myself, we are grateful to the real catalyst behind these books, our clients and patients, for the years of feedback that they have given us. There are too many to name, but each one was an important step in the development of these techniques.

Several of the original pictures and stories have been transferred over from my first book, and athletes I've worked with online have sent testimonials and photos to be included into the new books.

While our models, and the athletes who gave testimonials, aren't famous to the world, their stories are real – and without them these books would not exist.

My life has been blessed by all of the people I have just mentioned, and so many others. I hope you enjoy the books, and that the self-treatments bring you the benefits that others have experienced.

Yours in Health,

Julie Donnelly

Zev M. Cohen, M.D.

"When did you decide to become a doctor?" is a question I am often asked. My answer is always the same. It probably started when I was an infant in my mother's arms. She would show me off to her friends and say, "this is my son, he's going to be a doctor!"

Well, maybe that's not exactly how it happened. What is certain is the love and devotion my parents showed me while I was growing up. Not only did they teach me the importance of a good education, but also they instilled in me the values of honesty, caring, love, charity and compassion. Tools as necessary as a stethoscope for the daily practice of medicine.

My father taught me that I could do anything, if I try hard enough, and my mother taught me to think for myself and not follow the crowd. I am who I am because of who they are!

My gratitude to my loving parents goes beyond words. The feelings that I have, and carry with me every day of my life, are precious and for that I am forever grateful.

Not many years ago I was practicing medicine in a busy Internal Medicine office. I practiced by "the book", the way I had been taught in my medical school and residency training. But in my heart I knew there was a lot more to the practice of medicine. Medical textbooks didn't have all the answers!

I met Julie Donnelly at a Charity Health Fair; our immediate connection was, I feel, divinely inspired. She opened my mind to an area of medicine that is glaringly missing from medical training: the area of treating muscles to relieve many types of acute and chronic conditions. This new understanding has dramatically changed the way I treat patients on a daily basis.

Together, we have been able to restore many people to good health, allowing people to be pain free – and many times we have rescued people from "the knife". Julie's techniques of treating muscles, called the Julstro System, has so effectively been able to treat conditions such as Carpal Tunnel syndrome, that surgery has been cancelled on countless occasions. Julie, as the quintessential teacher, has taught thousands of patients how to treat themselves. Not only are they pain free when they leave my office, but they are equipped with the knowledge of how to treat their condition, should it return. Her tireless energy, strong focus, and never-ending enthusiasm are what keep both the Carpal Tunnel Treatment Center, and Julstro Muscular Therapy Center, going strong. I can't thank her enough.

My family, friends, and office staff, are all collectively a part of this book. I have always considered us a team – each member of the team vitally important.

And, of course, I must thank the Creator of our wonderful universe – whose Pure and Good Energy is what keeps us all going!

Zev M. Cohen, MD

INTRODUCTION

You have decided that you need to take an important aspect of your well being into your own hands – wise move!

Years of experience with thousands of individuals; athletes, "weekend warriors" and "couch potatoes", has proven to us that muscle spasms are a primary cause of muscle pains and joint pains. We have seen people run from one doctor to another to get an answer – and still be in pain. They have gone to physical therapy, massage therapy, chiropractic, and taken medication by the truckload, and still the pain persists. Why?

The answer will become crystal clear as you read this book. Muscle spasms are the major culprit to the vast majority of joint and muscle pains.

Why You Need This Book

Every day you do the same movements over and over. They may be at work, or while you are relaxing. Exercise will certainly stress your body, pushing it beyond its limits! It also causes the muscles to suffer from repetitive strain injury, causing pain, often severe pain that prevents you from living your life as you choose.

When joint pain develops you are told to use RICE – "Rest, Ice, Compression and Elevation". But – YOU DON"T WANT TO REST! Exercise is your lifeblood; it is what makes you thrive. That is why we wrote *The Pain-Free Runner* – to keep you moving and pain-free!

What To Do If Your Area of Pain Is Not In This Book

The Pain-Free Runner is part of a series of Pain-Free sports books. This book focuses on those areas which most commonly affect runners; however, runners also do other sports and work as well, and as such, there are a whole host of other aches and pains that may be caused by other activities.

There is a Julstro™ *Pain-Free Triathlete* book that includes a treatment for every indicated area on the trigger point charts. If you don't find a relevant treatment for an area that is bothering you in this book, please go to http://www.julstro.com to find books that focus on other areas.

How This Book Is Organized

The Pain-Free Runner is divided into four parts:

Part I – Listening to the Wisdom of the Body
Part II – All You'll Ever Need to Know About Muscles and Joints
Part III – The Julstro Treatments
Part IV –Trigger Point / Muscle Charts and Glossaries

Part I – Listening to the Wisdom of the Body

Written by JoAnn Dahlkoetter, Ph.D., best-selling author of YOUR PERFORMING EDGE. JoAnn is an internationally recognized sports psychologist, past winner of the San Francisco Marathon and 2nd place finisher in the Hawaii Ironman Triathlon World Championship.

Part II – All You'll Ever Need to Know About Muscles and Joints

Read Part II thoroughly to understand the "why" and "how" of muscles. They are the cause of your pain, and knowing how they work will enable you to treat them properly and quickly.

Chapter 1, Our Magnificent Muscles
In this chapter you will receive the basics of muscle movement and why muscles will shorten. This is the key to the entire problem and can't be overlooked.

Chapter 2, The Basics: How A Joint Moves
This chapter builds on Chapter 1 information and answers many questions.

Chapter 3, Avoiding Needless Surgery: Backs, Knees, and Carpal Tunnel Syndrome

In this chapter we examine why muscles have been ignored when searching for the answer to joint and muscle pain. It takes a general look at conditions that can be easily reversed by simply finding and treating the muscle spasms, and then stretching the muscle back to its proper length. This chapter shows why muscles cause conditions that are typically not considered to be a muscular problem, such as carpal tunnel syndrome, rotator cuff, knee pain, and how you can stop it immediately.

Chapter 4, Prevent Injuries Through Proper Exercise

This chapter introduces a vital key to being a runner and staying pain-free. Avoiding problems in the first place should be your personal goal. This chapter focuses on an Introduction to Physiology of Exercise and is written by Shawn Boom. An Ironman Triathlete himself, Shawn is an Exercise Physiologist and Personal Fitness Trainer for elite athletes.

Chapter 5, The Core Workouts for Fast Runners

This chapter offers you a training program that is well balanced and geared to preventing injuries while still maximizing your training program. This chapter is a natural "fit" in The Pain-Free Runner and completes the process of learning how to exercise at your optimum level – and stay well!

Chapter 6, The Julstro™ Method of Self-treatment

A complete explanation of the Julstro System is covered in this chapter. These will be your everyday "tools" to keep your muscles and joints healthy.

Chapter 7, The Trigger Point Charts

Trigger points are introduced, along with charts that are designed to help you locate the source of your pain. This chapter is the core of The Pain–Free Runner and is required reading to ensure that you use this book properly as a resource guide.

Part III – The Julstro Treatments

The thirteen chapters that make up this section of the book combine the areas shown in the trigger point charts with the Julstro self-treatments. Clear, easy-to-read text is complimented with photographs to help you to find and treat the spasms that are causing you pain. Each body part is individually covered.

Part IV –Trigger Point / Muscle Charts and Glossaries

On the trigger point charts you locate where you are feeling the pain – and you will find where the true source of that pain can be found. The spasm is often far from the area of discomfort, in fact, it may even be on the opposite side of your body!

The logic is simple to follow when using these charts. After you locate the area of pain on the referenced Trigger Point Chart, simply look up the muscle that is listed in the Table of Contents. You will be directed to the treatment for that muscle.

The muscle charts show you the details of the muscle connections, which help you to understand why you can feel pain in area distant from the spasm.

Where to Go From Here

Take a minute to glance through the book, getting comfortable with what's inside. Read Part One thoroughly, then start to relieve the pains that are holding you down.

Is it possible to be a runner, and be pain-free?

YOU BET IT IS!!

PART I: LISTENING TO THE WISDOM OF THE BODY

By JoAnn Dahlkoetter, Ph.D.

Learn to hear the whispers of the body and mind before they have to shout

An athlete came into my office a month ago complaining that, "Whenever an important race comes up something goes wrong, either mentally or physically. I can't seem to pull it all together when it really counts. I seem to be counterproductive, self-defeating, and continually sabotaging myself." I hear this type of complaint from athletes across the board, regardless of what sport or what level of play. For example, running can be such a challenging sport that requires so many bones, muscles, and connective tissue to work well together, it's easy to misjudge the body's limits and create an injury.

In team sports we're often taught by coaches to not pay too much attention to aches and pains. We are told: "Don't be a wimp – just get through the work out. We have a race this Sunday." So we often ignore the subtle symptoms. We prod on, making sure we complete our designated weekly mileage, doing a small amount of tissue damage each day, until our body screams for attention. Once an injury sets in, the healing and recovery then takes much longer than if we had learned to pay attention each day.

Sports Car Mentality

The body in fact has critical information for us. We need only to listen carefully, sense its soft messages, and follow its direction regularly. We need to first check in with our bodies before blindly moving ahead with our training plan. Indeed, **to train consistently and to stay healthy, we need to treat and care for our bodies like a finely tuned sports car.**

Over the next month I worked with the athlete described above. I showed him a technique involving listening and dialoguing where he learned to tune in to his body and mind with a sense of compassion and curiosity. In fact he launched into a journey that led to profound and lasting change in his running, which then carried over to the rest of his life. I have used this dialoguing technique successfully with so many athletes that it is well worth incorporating into your training plans. The process does not take extra time, only a greater awareness during the time you are training.

What I'm proposing here is a body-oriented process of awareness and healing. You can learn a method of sensing how you feel – physically and mentally. Then you can have a dialogue with your feelings and sensations where **you** do most of the **listening.** Athletes tend to be action-oriented, driven, and goal-directed. **They are accustomed to actively telling their bodies what to do - most of the time not so tactfully.**

You may say to yourself: "Pick up the pace, you slug, your shoulders are too stiff, why aren't you catching that guy in front of you?" What do you do when an uncomfortable feeling develops in your body (e.g. calf cramping or knee aching)? The typical reaction is to try to over-ride it. Perhaps you yell at it a bit: "Why does this stupid pain have to come on right now, when I've got 13 miles to go in the marathon?" Or you might beat yourself up mentally: "If only I had trained harder, my knee wouldn't freeze up like this."

Becoming Quiet and Listening

What does not occur to most athletes is to become quiet and to listen to the body's sensations. The key to preventing injury is to let your body give you this crucial feedback, especially while warming up for your regular workouts. Then you can take in and respect its wisdom before deciding on your course of action.

When you let the body speak, you are allowing yourself to be open to the depth and richness of your whole self – body, mind, and spirit. Once you pay attention to a sensation (e.g. tension or pain), it is more likely to release, and let you go on with your training in a more clear, and focused way. You'll also gain a better sense of what you need to do, if anything, to help the body function more efficiently (e.g. alter your posture, training form, breathing, etc.). Often we don't need to change anything at all. The body can heal and correct itself. **Awareness alone can often take care of the problem.**

Have you ever wondered during workout, "Am I doing the right thing for my body today? Should I be going this far, or this fast when I'm just returning from an injury? Is this workout helping to strengthen that area, or is it further aggravating the tendons that are still weak and vulnerable? Am I ready to take my training to the next level, or should I be conservative and stay with the same workouts for another week?" Regular listening and dialoguing with the body, as I will describe below, can fully answer all these questions, and give you a strong sense that you are doing the right thing.

Consulting With Your Body

It is now well accepted that we can confer with our bodies to assess if we are eating the proper food and if we are getting enough sleep. We understand that our bodies know what it feels like to be in good health, and what it's like when we're on the edge of a cold or flu, or injury. We know the positive sensations of having energy to spare and being very focused. We also know when we've let ourselves become way too tired or let our bodies get torn down.

Indeed, **we understand how to recognize the extreme states, but what about the subtle stages in between?** With arduous training and regularly challenging the muscles and tissues to work harder, we are continually tearing the body down. And don't forget, the mind is also challenged and needs recovery. This repair and healing process is going on constantly, for both the body and mind. The question is what are you doing to be more aware, and to facilitate that healing process?

Our bodies are wise in many ways beyond what is acknowledged by the average person. They can show us the path to optimal health and fitness if we so choose. Our bodies carry knowledge not only about how we are training, but how we are treating ourselves, what we value and believe, how we have been hurt emotionally, and how we are living our lives. Have you ever noticed when you think about that coach or parent who mistreated you, the pain in your neck or shoulder gets worse? Our bodies know which people are good for us to train with and which ones deplete and degrade us. And our physical selves know the best path to move up to the next level in our performance.

Below I have described a technique of tuning in and listening to the body in a caring, non-judgmental way that can save you months of time being on the injured list. Using this technique of listening and dialoguing can become a window into this expansive domain of knowledge that is accessible through the body. This type of work allows you to hear the soft warnings of the body and mind before they have to scream for attention. Then you'll be on your way to remaining healthy throughout the year.

Benefits of Listening to the Body

What kinds of problems best lend themselves to this sort of technique?

- Athletes who are training hard but feel stuck can use this listening technique to get their training moving again. You may be wondering: "I keep doing the same workouts, but the progress isn't there. There's something I'm not understanding about my body and my training."

- Some athletes may need to work on a problem with an addiction (e.g. overeating, drinking, caffeine, drugs). This technique can help release you from the power of your addiction by allowing you to listen carefully to the part of you that is responsible for the addictive behavior, and gain its cooperation.

- Athletes who have difficult or overwhelming feelings can learn to have a better relationship with their emotions. Strong feelings (anger, fear, sadness) can sometimes wash over us like ocean waves, and they can interrupt effective training. However, these emotions are there for a reason. They have an important message to convey. They bring back an important part of our wholeness. We need to learn to listen to their story without becoming overwhelmed. With this technique, you can begin to have a comfortable relationship with strong feelings, and acknowledge them without being drowned by them.

- Competitive athletes often have a highly critical side that makes training less enjoyable. You may want to quiet your critical side and enhance self-acceptance. With practice, you can turn your inner critic into an ally and supporter. Once you accept all parts of yourself (e.g. even the part that sometimes gets injured) this will allow deeper and more meaningful improvement in your training.

Creating an Atmosphere of Trust

Before beginning the work of listening to the body, we need to first establish a safe, trusting environment for communication. Imagine for a moment that you are walking along a trail, and you notice a small bashful animal peeking out from behind a tree. The animal is not a danger to you, but you would like to help it feel safe and relax around you. How would you accomplish this? What atmosphere would you like to create? You certainly would not run toward it shouting. You would probably be still and patient, or move very slowly and gently. You would be interested in it, watching carefully for signs that it feels comfortable around you. You would notice when it might be all right to move in a little closer.

The technique of dialoguing with your body described below is a process of listening to something inside yourself that wants to communicate with you. Just like getting to know the shy animal, your body may first need to establish that you are trustworthy, that you have created a safe place for it to deliver its message. So you need to create a safe, non-judgmental environment to do this work. Now you're ready to try this exercise.

Awareness Exercise #1 – Being in touch with your Body:

Take a moment and notice what you are feeling right now in your body or mind. If you are working out, notice if you have any nagging pain. Is it possible to simply let the feeling be there without trying to change it? Just notice how you are in this moment and say: "Yes, this is how I feel". Or say to the uncomfortable sensation: "Yes, I know you're there". You may have a tendency to judge your body as soon as you notice any discomfort and say, "I shouldn't be feeling this way". Or you may try to analyze your body pain saying: "Why do I always feel this way? Why doesn't my body perform like I want it to?" None of these ways are effective in helping the situation. This usually creates more body tension and discomfort.

However, when you allow your bodily sensations to be as they are and just acknowledge them, then they can change for the better on their own. When they are allowed just to be, they can settle down to have a conversation with you, and that conversation leads to positive change. You can really tune in and understand what your symptoms are telling you.

I utilized this exercise with one of my athlete clients who was experiencing hamstring pain while training for an ice dancing competition. After acknowledging the sensation she noticed an immediate sense of physical relief. She said: "The sensation is still there, but it's no longer painful. Now that it has my attention, it doesn't need to hurt and nag at me anymore."

Awareness Exercise #2 – Dialoguing with your Body:

Once you've established an area of your body that you would like to work on, you can begin a dialogue. Ask yourself: "What bodily sensation am I most aware of? What part needs my attention?" Once you identify a certain area, then ask yourself: "What exactly does it feel like?" Find the right words to describe it. Make sure you have the best words to fully articulate how it feels (e.g. tight shoulders, heavy feet, mind racing, etc.) You can write these thoughts down in a journal later. Next, gently acknowledge its presence. You could say, for instance: "Yes, I know you're there." Rather than fighting with the body as we often do, saying, "Oh God, there's that darn knee pain again", this time you can simply notice the sensation with a quiet curiosity, and begin to learn about it. Then just notice what happens. Become aware of any change in the sensation.

Now you can begin asking that part of the body what it needs. Or you can ask: "What needs to happen next for it to get better?" You can learn, for instance, if it just needs your quiet company? Does it need more care and attention? Does it need some special treatment?

Next you could **ask your body to show you how "completely healed" would feel.** How would it feel to have the problem cleared up, resolved satisfactorily. The body knows now how it would feel to have the situation resolved, even though your analytical mind may have no idea how that could happen. Ask your body to show you by beginning to feel that way right now. That kind of suggestion helps create an opening for new ways of being and perhaps healthier ways of treating your body.

The body's solutions are infinitely better, more creative, and healthier than anything your logical mind can dream up. You may feel stuck, but your body isn't. Once you begin to listen, understand, and dialogue with your body, it will show you its ageless wisdom. It will let you in on its critical secrets for staying healthy and moving forward with your training. You can then train more consistently and remain healthy throughout the year. You'll gain a new level of sensitivity to the body that can take you to new performance highs.

JoAnn Dahlkoetter, Ph.D., author of YOUR PERFORMING EDGE, is an internationally recognized sports psychologist, past winner of the San Francisco Marathon and 2nd in the Hawaii Ironman Triathlon. To see her NEW BOOK and VISUALIZATION CD, visit www.YourPerformingEdge.com, *or call 650- 654-5500. Dr. Dahlkoetter provides coaching by phone for optimal mind-body performance. For a FREE NEWSLETTER with valuable training tips and articles, Email:* joann@YourPerformingEdge.com.

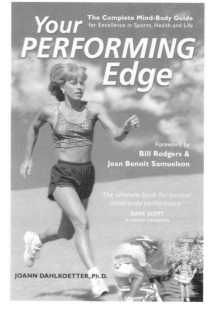

PART II: ALL YOU'LL EVER NEED TO KNOW ABOUT MUSCLES AND JOINTS

CHAPTER 1

Our Magnificent Muscles

Zev M. Cohen, MD

Our muscles comprise the largest part of our body. Indeed, they are the largest single organ of the body, and make up the bulk of its weight. All together, humans have about 300 paired-muscles, totaling approximately 600 muscles.

Each muscle, or muscle group, has its unique function. Some muscles work alone, others work together in unison. The amount of movements we possess, as a result of the combination of muscle fibers being utilized, are unlimited. Observe your hand and wrist, and the number of ways it moves, turns, twists, and so on. Despite all this movement, each muscle has only one function, i.e.: to contract or relax. As one muscle group contracts (shortens), an opposing muscle group relaxes (lengthens).

It's that simple…or is it?

An absolutely perfect symphony of movements must take place for each step we take. When you ate breakfast this morning, the muscles responsible for chewing had to contract, and relax, thousands upon thousands of times! In fact, to continue our example of breakfast, let's take a closer look at what was involved.

You used the muscles of your foot and toes, ankles, legs, thighs, and back, to go to the table and sit down. The muscles of your eyes, neck, shoulders, chest, arms, wrists, hand, and fingers were all in motion. And lastly, of course the muscles of the face, which are responsible for chewing and swallowing, were working constantly.

And what's most amazing is we didn't give it a single thought – it all "sort of" took place naturally!

The muscles of the human body are in use 24 hours a day, 7 days a week, 365 days a year. Despite this enormous amount of use, most of us spend little, or no, time caring for our muscles. Obviously, with such extensive and continued use, we must experience "wear and tear". In medical terms, this is known as Repetitive Strain Injury (RSI).

Let's face it; we are all creatures of habit. Which means we tend to do the same things in the same way, over and over again. The way I brushed my teeth this morning was exactly the same way I brushed them before bedtime. That goes for yesterday, the day before, and probably the last 10-20 years. The way we sit, stand, walk, drive, read a book, exercise, work at a computer – and any other movement – are all-important elements to the condition of our muscles.

Whether you are a homemaker or a construction worker... a typist or an interstate trucker... a musician or an electrician...the stress and strain placed on your muscles, each and every day, is enormous!

Repetitive Strain Injuries, or "wear and tear", tend to occur most often when muscles are used repeatedly, the more strength used, the more stress is placed on the muscle. However, you do not need to be moving to be using a muscle!

While quietly sitting and reading a book, although seeming relaxed, the muscles of the fingers, hands, and arm are all in use. The same goes for the neck and back muscles. It's ironic, isn't it, that you can be the victim of Repetitive Strain Injury while quietly sitting in your easy chair, reading a book! In fact, sitting is a very common cause of low back pain, because it contracts a muscle called the psoas. The more force exerted, the longer the time the muscle group is in use, and the less time spent on relaxing, and stretching, are all important factors to muscle injury.

Sometimes it's obvious: you mowed the lawn or shoveled snow from the walk, or started an aerobics class, and the next day you are sore, or maybe you had low back pain the day after lifting your child. These are simple cause and effect injuries. However, very often it is much less obvious - a contracted muscle in the neck or chest might cause pain and discomfort to the wrist and hand, which are the symptoms of carpal tunnel syndrome, but there isn't any pain in the neck or chest. This is known as "referred pain".

In the 1960's, Janet Travell, MD, conducted research that proved that muscle spasms caused pain to be felt in areas far from the spasm. She called the spasms "Trigger Points". Muscles often cause many–previously not well-understood– illnesses, such as: fibromyalgia, tinnitis (ringing in the ears), headaches, TMJ (jaw pain), many arthritic conditions, joint pains, tennis elbow, sciatica, and carpal tunnel syndrome!

To understand why a muscle causes pain, it is necessary to have a basic understanding of the anatomy of muscles. A muscle has two ends; at each end there is a covering of connective tissue called a tendon. Each tendon connects to a bone, usually crossing a joint. When a muscle contracts, one bone remains stationary and forms a fixed point, the other end pulls the bone to make the joint move.

For example, let's look at the flexor muscle group, the thick muscles on the underside of your forearm. One end of the flexor muscles attaches to the arm near the inside of your elbow. The other end inserts onto your wrist, hand and fingers. When the flexors are relaxed your hand is open. When the flexors contract, it shortens and you can see, or feel, the muscle thicken your forearm. The shortening of the flexor cause your hand to curl into a fist, and your fist to move toward your arm.

The basic unit of a muscle is a single fiber. These individual fibers are grouped together to form a bundle of muscles. Each individual muscle fiber operates according to the "all or nothing" principle. This means that when the muscle fiber is stimulated, it will contract with all its force, it will not stop in the middle of the contraction. There is no middle of the road with a muscle; it is all – or nothing!

In reality, and under certain adverse conditions, muscle fibers might contract and remain "stuck" in the contracted position. This may cause an acute pain, such as a muscle spasm, or a cramp, which can be severe.

Usually, however, the results of shortened muscle fibers are more subtle. For example, shortened muscles might be the cause of someone's "hunch back", chronic headache, or carpal tunnel syndrome!

CHAPTER 2

The Basics: How a Joint Moves and Other Interesting Info

A muscle crossing over a joint gives that joint the ability to move. Movement of a joint is a two-step process: one muscle must contract and shorten while the opposing muscle must relax and lengthen.

When a spasm occurs in the muscle, the pain is usually felt at the insertion of the muscle (the place where the muscle attaches to the bone), which is at the joint. In the case of the biceps, the insertion is on the inside of your elbow on the lower portion of your arm, while the insertion of the triceps is just below the point of your elbow, so spasms in either of these muscles will most likely cause elbow pain.

While the contract/stretch rule is the process of every muscle throughout the body, for demonstration purposes we will show how the biceps muscle (A) and the triceps (B) work together.

To open your arm, the biceps must stretch (A) and the triceps must contract/shorten (B).

When the biceps contract (A) and the triceps stretch (B) the arm bends at the elbow.

motion

In order to be able to completely bend or straighten the arm, these muscles must both be able to contract and stretch fully. If, for example, the biceps contract and the triceps do not stretch, the restricted triceps will stop the movement and you will not be able to fully bend your arm.

The ankle joint is controlled by several muscles.

When the tibialis anterior (A) contracts it lifts your toes from the ground.

Meanwhile the calf muscles and Achilles tendon (B) must stretch.

In your calf you have two primary muscles with the Latin names: gastrocneimus (commonly called "gastroc"), and soleus. The "gastroc", originates above the knee, so it also assists at bending your knee; the soleus originates in the middle of the calf. They both go into the tendon in the back of your ankle, called the Achilles tendon, and then continue on to insert on the back of your heel.

When the calf muscles are contracted they pull on the Achilles tendon, which then pulls on the heel, allowing you to "push off" with your toes (B). To make this movement the tibialis anterior must stretch (A).

Under the primary calf muscles, there are also lesser known muscles which do not go into the Achilles tendon. These include the tibialis posterior, flexor digitorum longus and flexor hallucis longus. A spasm will cause pain in this area, making one think there is a problem with the Achilles tendon.

A muscle spasm, or contracted muscle, will cause pain at the insertion point of the muscle. This is known as referred pain. We use the following example to clearly illustrate this situation: if you pull your hair at the end, it hurts at the scalp where it inserts. It is the same with muscles. If you contract (pull) the bulk of the muscle (known as the belly of the muscle), it will hurt where the muscle inserts into the bone. When your calf muscles are contracted, they may hurt directly on the muscle. However, since it is pulling on the insertion, your heel may hurt – even when you aren't feeling anything in the calf!

Another phenomenon attests to the wisdom of the body. As the muscle is pulling the tendon away from the bone, the body sends bone cells to secure the attachment. As these bone cells collect, you get what is called a "spur", or a bump of bone. This is frequently seen at the heel and at the shoulder. To try to break down the spur without releasing the muscle tightness first is fruitless. The body's intelligence will simply send more bone cells to secure the tendon.

Stretching is vital to the movements of joints. A stretch works best when it is only done to the degree that it feels good, (you'll always know where that is), and is held for one full minute. We have seen people exercise – some to excess – but they rarely stretch sufficiently.

That is what this book is all about: using the Julstro System to release the tight spasms and contractions, and stretch your muscles. When you release a spasm you are also lengthening the muscle – it's like untying a knot and the rope gets longer.

Sprains Affect on Muscles

When you sprain a joint, for example the ankle, the muscles are suddenly overstretched, and then quickly released, causing multiple spasms to form in the muscle. Since a muscle is normally held in perfect tension, from the origination to the insertion, these spasms will cause a stress to be placed on the insertion point of the muscle at the joint, causing pain that will not cease until the spasms are released.

A sprain at any joint requires treatment of the spasms found in each muscle that crosses that joint. After the spasms are treated stretching will relieve the tension on the joint.

Broken Bones Effect on Muscles

When the bone breaks the muscle suddenly contracts totally. As the bone is set the muscle is pulled into place, but rarely are the muscle spasms treated to bring the fibers back to their correct length.

This results in the bone being strained by the multiple spasms that have formed during the sudden contraction. We have seen clients who have experienced pain for years after a bone break, even though the bone has healed perfectly. As soon as the muscle spasms are treated the pressure is removed from the bone, and pain is eliminated.

CHAPTER 3

Avoiding Needless Surgeries!

Through the years we have had countless numbers of clients come to our offices with severe joint pain. Many times they had already been thru a wide assortment of therapies without finding relief, and had then been scheduled to have surgery. On many occasions they didn't even come to us about the joint problem, they were there for other reasons and just "happened to mention it" to one of us. As you read this book you will find several examples of people who were heading for needless surgery – and were "spared the knife" by using the Julstro method of deep muscle therapy.

Of course, there are times when only surgery will help. When a tendon or ligament has been severed, only re-attaching the pieces will give pain relief and return mobility.

When you read Chapter 1, Our Magnificent Muscles, you gained an understanding of how muscles cause joint pain; therefore, we will only include a brief explanation here. Muscles insert at a joint, and when the muscle contracts the joint moves. However, when the muscle is in spasm it continues to contract, even when you are trying to move the joint in a different direction. Just as pulling your hair will cause you pain where it inserts at the scalp, so does pulling a tight muscle cause pain where it inserts at the joint. In his book "What You Don't Know Can Hurt You…Seven Important Facts about Carpal Tunnel Syndrome", Dr. Cohen has explained: "medical doctors aren't trained in how pain is caused by muscles. This is a major gap in understanding the body, and in pain management."

This is the case whether it is the quadriceps muscles that inserts at the knee, the calf muscles that insert at the Achilles tendon and the heel, the triceps muscle that inserts into the elbow; or any of the muscles of the forearm that insert into the wrist and hand. There have been innumerable surgeries done on joints that could have been avoided if only the muscles had been treated and lengthened.

When the muscles of the body cross over a nerve, such as the sciatic nerve in the buttocks, a spasm in the muscle will cause pain and numbness to be felt far from the spasm. In the case of the sciatic nerve the pain/numbness is felt in the hip, hamstrings, calf and arch of the foot.

While the problem occurs throughout the entire body, this is clearly understood by using wrist pain as an example. When a person is having pain in the hand and wrist, and numbness in the fingers, he may be misdiagnosed as having "carpal tunnel syndrome". This problem of misdiagnosis warrants further explanation.

Carpal Tunnel Syndrome is the #1 repetitive strain injury (RSI) in the USA, accounting for an estimated 400,000 carpal tunnel release surgeries in 2001. Tragically, many of these surgeries could easily have been avoided!

As we mentioned earlier, using the hair-pulling example, if you pull your hair your scalp will hurt. Don't "fix the scalp, let go of the hair. Carpal tunnel is exactly the same situation. Don't operate on the tunnel, simply let go of the muscles that are causing a strain at the tunnel – or at any point along the length of the median nerve.

Carpal Tunnel Syndrome occurs when the nerve in the wrist and hand (called the median nerve) becomes entrapped. The fact is, if the median nerve is entrapped anywhere along its entire length, one may experience wrist/hand pain and numbness. This is the vital piece that is being overlooked by most practitioners.

Since 95% of the median nerve is not in the carpal tunnel, it is safe to surmise that 95% of the potential source of the pain and numbness is not coming from within the tunnel. Therefore 95% of the surgery is unnecessary – *that would total 380,000 needless surgeries in 2001!*

The same can be said for knee surgery, low back surgery, and ankles.... the list goes on! Muscles are a serious missing piece in the pre-surgical treatment process. In the chapter on the shoulder, you will read that a spasm in the infraspinatus muscle will give the same symptoms as bursitis of the shoulder, and can also mimic the pain of a torn rotator cuff; the chapter on the leg shows how a spasm in the quadriceps will cause searing pain to be felt in the knee. However, surgery is NOT the answer – only releasing the muscle spasms will relieve the pain!

In order to stop the pain in your hand, and numbness in your fingers, to continue working and enjoying your life to the fullest, and to <u>avoid potential surgery,</u> it is important to understand the anatomy of the Carpal Tunnel. We suggest you visit our website so you may view the graphics demonstrating each step of this explanation.

There are 8 small bones in the wrist called the "carpal bones". These bones form the base of the carpal tunnel. A ligament called the Flexor Retinaculum, also known as the Transverse Carpal Ligament, forms the roof of the tunnel, commonly called "the bridge". Lay the back of your hand on a table, and look at this graphic.

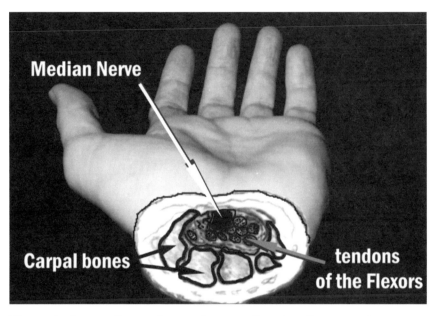

Through the small carpal tunnel passes the nine flexor tendons, along with the median nerve.

Any pressure exerted onto this area will squeeze the median nerve and cause pain and numbness to the hand and wrist.

For example: repetitive wrist or hand motions, such as working at a computer terminal, playing a musical instrument, sports, or even knitting, will cause swelling in the carpal tunnel.

To complicate things, the median nerve, which starts in the neck and travels down the arm to the wrist and hand, can become entrapped anywhere along its path by any of the muscles that cross over it. A pinched nerve in the neck, or anywhere along the path of the median nerve, may cause you to have pain in your hand. A simple analogy will demonstrate this point: A telephone line a few blocks away, when knocked down after a storm, may cause static on your telephone. This concept is exactly what happens when the median nerve is pressed on, or irritated anywhere along its entire path, a static message is sent to the muscle.

If you have access to a computer you can click on http://www.aboutcts.com/median_nerve.html to view the median nerve. This is the nerve that will cause pain and numbness to be felt in the chest, the upper back, the entire arm and also the hand.

The first muscle that may impact on the median nerve is the scalenes, which originate on your cervical (neck) vertebrae and insert onto the first rib.

When the scalenes are contracted by a spasm, they put pressure directly onto a bundle of nerves called the brachial plexus. This causes a multitude of problems, including numbness in the thumb and first two fingers.

The median nerve continues through the chest, arm and into the hand. Each of the following links will describe another part of the condition that is being labeled carpal tunnel syndrome – and are actually repetitive strain injuries of the various muscles.

As you read the text that is associated with the graphics, you will understand why you don't need carpal tunnel surgery, you only need to release the spasms in the muscles that impact the median nerve! We recommend you click on each link to examine this problem in depth.

To read a clear description of a muscle that raises your arm click on www.aboutcts.com/pectoralis_minor.html. This muscle causes spasms to occur without pain being felt in the area of the spasm, and is a key muscle in the numbness felt in the thumb and fingers.

When a person holds their arm up for extended periods of time, or sleeps with their arm tucked under their head, it may cause hand pain and numbness that is commonly thought of as a symptom of Carpal Tunnel Syndrome. Frequently, because of this reason, people wake up during the night and have to shake out their hand.

Releasing the contraction and spasms in the pectoralis minor will return blood flow, and sensation, to the arm and hand. We teach our clients how to change their sleeping habits and keep their arm down during the night.

The median nerve continues to travel under the biceps. One of the branches of the biceps originates on the coracoid process and has the same impact on the median nerve as the pectoralis minor. When the biceps are in contraction they are pulling down on the coracoid process and trapping the nerve under the bone.

It then goes into the forearm where it is frequently trapped by the tight flexor muscles, as shown in http://www.aboutcts.com/flexor_muscles.html.

At the Carpal Tunnel Treatment Center we have found that it is vital to work out each individual spasm in the flexor muscles. Stretching is important, but unless the spasms are released, the muscles cannot be stretched sufficiently to release the strain on the tendons and you develop tendonitis, an inflammation of the tendons.

Most people have heard the term "tendonitis", but they don't realize how a muscle causes this condition.

An analogy we've found useful is to describe the muscle/tendon/bone connection like the system that automatically opens your garage door. The muscle is comparable to the motor of the system, the tendon, a strong fibrous band that connects a muscle to a bone, is like the cable that runs from the motor to the door, and the bone is like the garage door.

When the motor (muscle) is turned on, it pulls on the cable (tendon). The cable then pulls on the door (bone), and the door moves. Likewise, when the muscle pulls on the tendon, the tendon then pulls on the bone and the bone moves.

Look at http://www.aboutcts.com/flexor_muscles.html to view the muscles that enable you to close your hand into a fist and whose tendons pass through the carpal tunnel along with the median nerve.

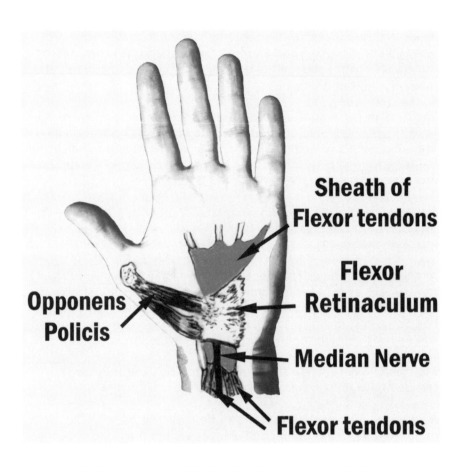

Sheath of Flexor tendons

Flexor Retinaculum

Opponens Policis

Median Nerve

Flexor tendons

The muscle that is responsible for drawing your thumb into the palm of your hand is the opponens pollicis. You can see the muscle, and the bridge by going to:
http://www.aboutcts.com/the_thumb.html.

The thick muscle at the base of the thumb is used millions of times a day. When this muscle is in spasm, it pulls down the roof of the Carpal Tunnel, and puts pressure on the median nerve.

When the flexor muscles, or the thumb muscles, are in spasm they put excessive pressure, or pull, on the carpal tunnel. Often this is tested by an EMG (Electromylogram). An EMG is an unpleasant test frequently used to diagnose Carpal Tunnel Syndrome. An electrode (needle) is placed into a nerve, and a second electrode is placed a distance away. An electrical charge is then passed between the two electrodes.

The technician measures the length of time it takes for the signal to go through the nerve, and if it is delayed you are told you have a "positive" EMG, confirming that you have carpal tunnel syndrome. And you do, but it is because the tendons have trapped the nerve within the tunnel.

At this point you have a few choices. A hand surgeon can cut open the wrist and snip the ligament of the carpal tunnel. However, a much easier approach, and far less painful, is to learn how to treat the spasms of the muscles we have just discussed. This will effectively stop the wrist/hand pain and numbness!

Overuse of anti-inflammatory drugs, and unnecessary surgery, is rampant throughout the USA, causing pain, paralysis, and even death! Dr. Cohen has written an informative book: What You Don't Know CAN Hurt You…7 Important Facts About Carpal Tunnel Syndrome, which you will receive free by going to: http://www.aboutcts.com and registering for the Carpal Tunnel Treatment Center newsletter.

You don't need to open the tunnel – you just need to release the pressure on the nerve!

As mentioned above, Carpal Tunnel Syndrome is the #1 Repetitive Motion Injury in the United States. If you continue doing the movements that are causing the condition, the problem will only get worse.

As you learn how to find and treat the spasms that are pressing on a nerve, you can rest assured that when the repetitive strain injuries of physical activity occur (and they will) anywhere in your body, you will be able to avoid surgery!

CHAPTER 4

Prevent Injuries Through Proper Exercise

By Shawn Boom

It was thirteen hours or so into a mountain biking race that I first noticed the fireflies.

With another twelve hours to go, I took a moment to get off my bike, virtually stopping the race, simply to take in the glowing field of stars on earth.

I was looking down the valley, which I had been biking up and down since noon and thinking how beautiful the 1:00 AM morning was turning out to be. Even through the salted and muddied vision I had earned though the rigors of the race, fireflies somehow became a symbol to me of the great payoffs hard work can lead us to, as athletes, and as people.

In the days preceding the race the butterflies filled my stomach and I was unable to eat. Nervous energy is a challenge for most athletes and it is no different for me. At that point, my last real meal was a few days ago and a combination of physical, emotional and nutritional exhaustion was becoming a near hallucinogenic bliss. Faced with challenges, and motivated by goals, athletes are poised to shine and when they do, the world becomes iridescent in their eyes – it is also this point that the fireflies start to flicker. Like the modern artists of today, this wasn't the first time I've brought myself to tears over the beauty of living life with fireflies as objectives - and it surely wouldn't be the last.

Over the past nine years I've been working hard to become the best person I can be. People choose to pursue the challenge of figuring out who they are in many different ways. So far, my path of self-discovery has taken me through four Ironman Triathlons, one-hundred or so short course triathlons, two 24+ hour cycling races, 19 marathons, a handful of adventure races, world famous rock climbs, volcano and mountain summits and through the ever important college degree (Exercise Physiology, of course). The one thing I have learned through all of these experiences is that the important part of being me is that I am able to share my love for adventure with other people. It is for this reason that I am very pleased to have found Julie Donnelly & Dr. Cohen, and the Julstro techniques. They are dedicated to helping athletes continue to shine by taking both a proactive, and rehabilitation, approach to injured people seeking their own personal fireflies.

I am currently employed by Balanced Body Inc. in the industry of Pilates. I live in Sacramento, California with my wife Bethany, and pug dog Killian. I have coached many people in their first pursuits in sports, and written some fun articles on training. I hope you enjoy the articles and rehab techniques you read in this book, and I welcome any and all comments, criticisms and curiosities.

Everyone has their own firefly; please keep looking for yours.

Shawn Boom

The Physiology of Exercise

Having been an athlete for my entire life, I seem to have acquired a great sense of taste for the adventures and discoveries sports have lent to me. The vagabond nature of my psyche has allowed me to try many different training tactics in pursuit of the highly sought after "fit body". I've done races lasting a matter of seconds…"Dad, I'll race you to the car", up to a matter of days "Hmmm, I guess I can handle sleep deprivation and malnourishment for extended periods of competition".

My point is that I have shaped my life after the pursuit of fitness. My college studies were in Exercise Physiology, I have partaken in endless laboratory experiments that drew blood, measured breathing and calculated power output. I have raced in many Ironman Triathlons, cycled longer than my behind cares to remember, climbed mountains at extreme altitude and fired through adrenaline crushing dares – all to find out how far the human body and mind can be pushed without falling apart.

What I have found by socializing with some of the countries great adventure seekers, and beginner exercises, is that all athletes need to continually learn and think about the inner-workings of their training program if they want to improve their fitness levels and mental attitude, diet, lifestyle factors, and racing seasons.

Many beginners have little concept about the reason they train, other than their personal trainer or coach tells them they really ought to do another set or a few more repetitions. Some long time athletes or "magazine-aholics" out there probably know the variable improvements the human body is capable of making on a biochemical and physiological level. There seems to be an unusual consensus in the fitness industry that knowing what happens to the human body under physical stress and recovery actually assists the body in the process. It is in my opinion that an athlete "doing what they are told" should really be "telling their body what it is going to do". That is to say, getting "in shape" is much easier to do when a person understands what exactly being "in shape" means.

What exactly is "Getting in Shape?"

"Exercise helps you look good naked"… it's a popular slogan many health clubs are using lately, suggesting that if we look good naked we will be "in shape". While changing our physique is often a by-product of exercise, it shouldn't be the prime focus of concern. In general, the human body is capable of reacting to various stimuli as needed.

If a couch potato doesn't offer much in the way of exercise for their body, the body won't offer much in the way of health for said person. If a runner demands that her body perform exercise six to seven days per week, the body will generally respond accordingly. The body's response to what we ask it to do is really where we can find the roots of exercise physiology. Getting in shape is about molding and changing the human body from all levels, beginning with broad changes in things such as our breathing and ending on very specific details like the manipulation of the smallest cellular composition comprehendible to science.

I've got a 'weekend warrior' friend who can model one process by which a hard trying runner gets in shape. Through his racing season, Rusty's body will undergo some very predictable and expected transformations, assuming the training program is put together by someone extremely brilliant and good looking (such as myself). Sometime in the middle of the spring thaw, Rusty knows that he should start training for the summer racing season. Like the good lad that he is, Rusty announces to his friends, "Pals, it's time I began training to increase my capillary functions, improve my ability for rapid fat oxidation, increase my ventilatory capacity, raise my VO2 max, decrease my resting heart rate, raise my lactate threshold,

speed my recovery, increase my lean muscle mass, decrease my..."
and Rusty's friend cuts him off saying "dude" (yes, Californians still
use the word 'dude') you mean you need to get in shape?"

Yes, Rusty is talking about a few of the things that we strive to do
when we athletes get in shape. Below you'll notice a list of some
things that change inside our bodies when we get "in shape". Think
about a typical training week for our weekend warrior runner
friend. Aside from the inherent garble of needless responsibilities
such as work, laundry, cleaning and family (that is a joke), Rusty is
going to give his body somewhere in the neighborhood of five to
ten training sessions per week.

Each training session can be quantitatively measured by different
things (frequency, intensity, time, sport) and assuming that Rusty's
program is laid out correctly, each session will focus on different
parts of his physiology, technique and mental toughness. The early
parts of the season will be tailored to facilitate physiological
adaptation while the middle season training will help him with
tuning motor skills and increasing biochemical activities in each
little cell. The later portion of Rusty's season will be used to
generate muscular power, speed and tapering, respectively.

The major things I encourage athletes to pay attention to in their
training are the things that can be measured frequently by
themselves that are as non-invasive as possible. Thankfully, exercise
labs are not a requisite to becoming a top-notch athlete. While
having an exercise physiologist or coach perform specific tests with
instruments of elaborate precision is almost always a beneficial
learning experience, there are inexpensive tools on the market
today that can give you great means by which to assess your current
"in-shapeness" as well as serve to be motivating tools.

There are many ways to express exercise intensity:

1. Calories over a given period of time
2. Absolute Power output
3. Perceived Exertion
4. Multiples of resting metabolic rate
5. Relationship of relative metabolic rate relating to Lactate
   Threshold
6. Relationship of relative metabolic rate relating to VO2 Max
7. Relative percentage of Maximum Heart Rate

Number seven from the above list, Heart Rate, is in my opinion the number one measurement for self coached athlete.

For people new to Heart Rate (Zone) Training, a heart rate monitor comes in two parts. The first part on modern day monitors is a transmitter, generally taking the form of a chest strap. The second part of the equation is a wristwatch that gathers electrical impulses sent from the transmitter and relates them into information called "Beats Per Minute (BPM)". This number is the amount of beats an athletes heart is beating per minute and in my estimation training with this number in mind is one of the single most accurate ways to get in shape. If you are an athlete without a heart rate monitor find a way to gain access to one – they are extremely economical today.

When am I officially in shape?

I hear this question all of the time. Generally it is presented to me in the form of a statement such as, "I need to lose ten pounds" with the inference being that the 10 extra pounds is really what is keeping that person from being in shape. Incidentally enough, the loss of those ten pounds (as described above) is simply a by-product of other changes occurring within the body. The starting point for beginner and elite athletes who want to perform to the best of their physiological abilities is to regularly document their workout measurements in a training log. There are a good number of computer software programs on the market for the tech-geeks, and there are double the amounts of great workout logbooks for sale in print. I simply use a plain printed calendar with a month and week view. Whatever your choice, arm yourself first with this calendar and an accompanying 3-ring binder folder. The binder will be used to collect articles, document test results, write down notes and tips, and collect whatever other useful tidbits you find. Remember, sports are just as much about the educational side of the game as they are the physical.

The human mind has proven over and again its capabilities to directly influence racing performance, training results and yes, aesthetic appearances (for you who haven't quite caught on to the whole point of this article yet). The real answer to the question "When am I officially in shape?" is that regardless of your current starting point, once you show that you are on a linear line of continual improvements, you are getting in shape! This line isn't just a theoretical; it is a positive line you can document in measurable terms.

General Fitness Assessment Tests

The first thing you need to do is assess your current physical condition. If you haven't worked out in the past 12 months, do yourself a favor and swallow your pride by visiting a doctor. Assuming you are healthy and ready to begin a training program (or begin training at a higher level, for you elites), you will need to learn your maximum heart rate. There are many ways to access tests offering this information. One of the greatest resources I can lend you to is my friend Sally Edwards. After finishing 16 Ironman Triathlons, Sally was inducted into the Triathlon Hall of Fame! Please take a few moments now and visit her website at http://www.Heartzones.com. While you are there, choose a protocol for calculating your max heart rate and get outside to take the test. Once you have that number written down in your 3-ring binder, revisit the tests below. If you don't currently have a heart rate monitor, please beg, borrow or steal one because a serious athlete cannot move forward without knowing their five heart rate zones. If you have any questions, contact staff@heartzone.com.

Armed with your max heart rate numbers, the next tests I will encourage you to take include:

* The Anaerobic Threshold
* The one-mile running heart rate test
* The 10 mile cycling heart rate test
* The recovery heart rate test

At the very least, you should build each of these tests into your training regime once each month. By continually monitoring the results (and ideally graphing them out in a computer spreadsheet program) you will become familiar with many of the changes your body is making while you train. When you have test results for the above five test, I'd say you're in pretty good shape already!

Remembering here that the goal of training is to develop stronger muscles, a healthier heart, better functioning joints, and an overall feeling of euphoria for life, spend some time listening to your body and how it reacts to the exercise you have given it today. Your body will, in turn, react to you in the way that you ask of it.

CHAPTER 5

The Core Workouts of Fast Runners

Shawn Boom

When I want to climb a mountain, I train by hiking, climbing and running and weight lifting the certain muscles I know I'm going to need during my big day. When I want to hit a baseball really far, I spend time working on my technique of swinging a bat and weight training specific muscle movements I know I'll need during the big game.

Likewise, when I want to compete fast (or just simply finish a race for that matter) I follow the principle of exercise called "sport specific training". This means that not only do I run and weight lift but I do them in a systematic and scientific approach so that on race day I can show up with confidence and a finely tuned body.

Sports specific training in means that the exercises and workout sessions an athlete does won't be of much benefit to the race unless it is either building strength for muscles or joints, helping with movement pattern training or conditioning the same metabolic pathways that will be used during the race itself. Keeping this principle in mind, the following is an infrastructure of a training program I use when training athletes I am coaching — as well as myself.

The Principle of Three

There are three essential workouts that occur in a regular training week for every advanced runner. Being that there are only a limited number of hours in a day, and unless you can take time off work, which I encourage if possible, many athletes hit the wall of life everyday. There comes a point, just like in races, that reality becomes the strongest beast inside the body and we can't go on with training unlimited amounts of time. When the garden hedges need cutting, the garage needs cleaning and the weekend is almost over, we all realize that there needs to be a concise and spelled out formula for getting and staying in shape. The three key workouts have been suggested by many before me and will be used by many after me. Nonetheless, utilizing these key workouts each week is a great goal to begin with.

THREE KEY WEEKLY WORKOUTS

Intervals

An interval is a repeat of low (easy effort) and high (hard effort) stress that results in the body's adaptation to a new and higher level of fitness. Interval training is a methodology of training that includes regular doses of low and high repeats of training.

Threshold workout

This workout is your favorite activity performed at moderate intensity. For me, it's a certain run I do down the river trail, or my morning bike ride that can be done easily before work. These workouts are moderate intensity, normally Zone 3 (70-80% MHR), and last about as long as the interval workouts ... but they're much easier.

Long workout

A long workout should be performed each week at a low intensity. For your long workouts, begin by doing one each week for 7 weeks. However long the long workout is, it should be based on time, not distance. Go at 70% for 7 weeks during this workout.

Take a look at your workout week. If you can't find each of these three types of workouts, tweak one of them to become one of these! Each of these workouts stresses your body a bit differently, teaching your cells and muscles to utilize different metabolic pathways, and helping you reach your goal in a systematic and effective manner.

The three-workout rule suggests that each week a runner will complete an "Interval", "Threshold" and "Long" workout.

This concept is based on the principles of adaptation and progression. As you become more fit, you can train at higher intensities and for longer periods of time using lower amounts of energy. By stressing the body in different ways, you are able to build a highly trained system of biological pathways that accommodate hard training efforts with the necessary physiological components as well as aid in healing when you train at lower levels.

Plateau

These workouts (long workout, threshold and interval workout) are all that is needed to help an athlete attain and maintain a certain level of fitness. Anything above and beyond these workouts is not necessary, though not necessarily harmful. A great runner can win races on this formula and a beginner will finish with incredible confidence by working her way up to this level. As progression and adaptation occur, athletes need to continue to change their training pattern (by varying there phases as discussed below and by including cross-training and weight lifting).

We can further break a training season down into four phases: Base, Speed, Power, and Peak. Depending on what point in the training season an athlete is, the time and intensity of these workouts will vary greatly.

A reasonable training cycle for a beginning runner would allow for 4 – 6 weeks of base training, 3 weeks of speed training, little or no time spent in power training and about 1 week spent "peaking". See the sidebar for more details on this terminology. This means that a beginner would need to start training no less than 8 weeks prior to their first race. I also don't recommend that beginners jump into a race that exceeds their longest training workout by 2 times. This means that if the longest workout a new runner has finished is one hour, then a race lasting longer than 2 hours should be reconsidered.

Four Phases of Training

While training theories differ throughout the world, the reoccurring theme infers that cycling the training doses is the most effective way to condition one's body to perform at a high level. Keeping in mind that "high level" is a relative term and that finishing a race might be a high level to one person and a simple expectation to another. The following are four general categories of training cycles I use when putting together all athletes training programs. The time allotted to each phase of training is a general statement and is transient based on past training experience. In addition, the following recommendations are based on portions of my personal experience as a triathlon coach and athlete, and represent my training philosophy, which has been shaped by a great number of teachers and researchers.

Base Training

2-8 weeks: Training done for longer periods of time at lower intensities. If measuring with a heart rate monitor, it is recommended that those in the base training phase train no higher than 70% of their max heart rate. Base training helps with anatomical adaptation including the strengthening of tendons and ligaments, increasing the red blood cell count, helping the body appropriately burn the correct combination of fats and carbohydrates, and much more.

Speed Training

2-4 weeks: After the base building phase, an athlete is generally overtaken with boredom and a strong desire to "go faster". Because 70% of max heart rate (MHR) is usually a slow pace for most athletes, speed training comes as a great relief and a welcome change. The first few weeks of speed training should concentrate on building strength more than speed. I generally like to spend 2 weeks doing ? of the amount of intervals I plan on accomplishing at the end of the speed session. For example, if I'm allowing my body 4 weeks of speed training by which at the end I plan on running 6 x 1 mile repeats at 85% MHR, I will spend the first two weeks building up from 3 or 4 miles at 80-85% MHR followed by some sports specific weight lifting (with repetitions of about 12-15).

I allow my body adequate base building and strength adaptation periods because I know my muscles are capable of getting stronger a lot faster than my tendons and ligaments. After a few weeks of light speed/strength training, my muscles are probably adapting and growing but my joints will lag behind a little bit. By slowing growing into the speed training, I am certain that I won't be hurt when it comes time to train hard. There is a tendency to go faster than necessary at an early point in the season and it can be detrimental to your training and life if you don't follow the principles of adaptation and progression. When beginning the speed-training phase, always pay close attention to the small changes and warning signals your body gives. If you feel a new "twinge" or a muscle that just "doesn't feel right", take a day or two completely off – because a few days of self treatment beats a few months of inactive living on the couch!

Power Training

2-3 weeks: Beginning runners will want to avoid this training phase of 3 weeks if they don't have previous experience with high intensity training. Advanced runners can use this phase for no more than three weeks without planning a new recovery cycle. The power workouts can do incredible harm to the muscular anatomy of a person who isn't well adapted. For this reason, I recommend that anyone planning to enter the power phase of training cycle through 2 speed phases (3 weeks each with one week recovery between) in order to adapt and progress to a point where injury can hopefully be avoided and at worst be limited. Power workouts for runners include moderate time investments with maximum power output.

Running on hills, cycling on a wind-trainer so as not to be interrupted by traffic, swimming high volume intervals and lifting more weights with less reps are included in the power training phase. Efforts last anywhere from 3 minutes in the pool to 10 minutes on the bike to 6 minutes running. Heart rates will exceed 93-95% MHR and adequate dietary intake is a must. If a beginner athlete wishes to skip the power phase, they can either choose to recycle through another speed phase (not changing intensity but adding time) or altogether advance to the peaking phase.

In the power phase, the adaptation and progression concept plays out in an obvious manner. By progressively lowering the number of reps or intervals and raising the intensity level or weights, the body is forced to do greater amounts of work output. Providing that there is a substantial recovery period between each hill, repeat or lift, the body will be capable of performing repeated exercises at highly intense levels. It is important to remember the principles of the nine-workout rule – just because this is the power phase doesn't mean that every workout is done as a power workout. The concepts of nine key workouts still applies, this phase just means that when intervals are part of a workout, they are done as outlined by the principles of power training. It is also important to note that the body doesn't get stronger while performing exercise; it actually breaks down while training.

The building up of our muscles and cells occurs in the times of our lives when we are recovering, such as sitting at our desk in the office, sleeping and stretching. When training at high levels, be sure to give intense rest periods to your body as well. Think of rest like a supplemental vitamin that aids in recovery. It is especially important to self-administer precautionary treatments to the body's muscles and cells. Eating good food is always important but having the correct balance when training in the power phase is highly related to muscle and joint recovery. Massage is always a good tool of injury prevention, as are proactive thermal treatments of contrasting temperatures.

Peaking

1 - 2 weeks: The peak training phase is where you can fine-tune your body and your equipment. About 2 1/2 weeks before the major race of the season, take in your last long workout. In the middle of the long workout, if you feel inspired, throw in some moderate intervals that slowly raise your heart rate by 10% of your race pace, lasting from 10 to 15 minutes. In the two weeks immediately after your last long workout, cut your workout time down to 45 minutes for beginners and no more than 1 hour and 15 minutes for Marathon Runners. During these last workouts, take a lot of recovery time and low heart rate training with the intermixing of some speed training, equivalent in intensity but less time that where you ended in the last speed phase of your training. This is the time when you should feel light on your feet, anxious and full of energy.

A well peaked athlete often gets crabby because the volume of training they are used to is cut back up to 50% and the usual energy outlet that once existed is no longer a viable option. There will be more time available in a runners day when she is peaking and I recommend doing light stretching and spending extra down time partaking in mind-body exercises.

Don't do anything "new" for exercise in the peaking phase. Plan to be "in shape" for yoga, Pilates, or whatever other supplemental training regimes you plan to use while peaking. I had a friend injure himself during the final training sessions prior to a big race simply because with a decrease in training volume he got bored and started playing softball for fun. The last time he had swung a bat was in high school and his triathlon was a miserable experience because he got to know the meaning of back spasms! During the Peaking phase, spend time concentrating on the race and enjoying time with your family – don't try anything new!

A Closer Look at the Key Weekly Workouts

The Long Workout

The purpose of the long workout each week is to develop and maintain a "base" as it is commonly referred to. Having a base is almost as elusive as being "in shape". There is no checkpoint by which one can determine they either have or have not established a base. Using the continuous measurement system outline in the above tests, one can, however, determine the movements of their physiological patterns and be able to study their own body's reaction to training doses.

In addition to working on an athlete's base, a long workout provides the joints and bones an opportunity to get used to working for a long time and offers the adequate time for building a stronger infrastructure.

The Threshold Workout

Of the many thresholds in an athlete's life, there are two very important ones to consider in the threshold workout. The first is called the aerobic threshold and generally falls between 50-55% of one's maximum heart rate. Workouts below this intensity are not really considered to be "workouts". That said, there are numerous benefits to training inside the aerobic workout, such as increased ability for tendons and ligaments to adapt to exercise before stressing them in harder workouts. Other benefits arise in the form fuel usage. It is in the aerobic threshold workouts that a person burns the highest percentage of fat as a fuel source.

Because through a complex series of chemical reactions, fat needs oxygen present (80-85% of the total calories burned here are fat calories).

The Interval Workout

By introducing interval training into a weekly workout regime, athletes become aware of many benefits not fully realized by regular training. While all athletes can derive benefit from interval training, I recommend that only experienced athletes partake in any intervals that take their heart rate over 90% of maximum. Intervals mean that training intensities vary in incremental units based on time, distance or a combination thereof. Common ways to denote intervals in a training program (and the way I use in this book) are as follows:

What the Workout Says	What the workout Means
4 x 1 mile @ 87% MHR on with 1.5 times rest	4 intervals of 1 mile each. Each interval is done at an effort of 807% of one's individual max heart rate. Whatever time the athlete finished the miles should be multiplied by 1.5 to determine rest time
8 x 1000 meters @ 90% MHR with 3 minutes recovery or to 65% MHR	8 intervals of 1000 meters each, performed at 90 percent of one's maximum heart rate. Time is not the determining factor in this kind of workout ~ recovery (measured by heart rate) is the indicator flag to watch. When an athlete finishes one of these intervals, they are free to begin the next immediately when their heart rate recovers to 65% of maximum heart rate.

Example: Running Interval Workout

	Intervals	Endurance	Anaerobic Threshold
Example Workout	4 x 1 mile @ 87%+ MHR with equal or 1.5 times recovery	8-15+ miles @ 60-70% MHR depending on distance of last long run	8 x 1000 meters at 90% MHR with 3 minutes recovery
Training Benefit	Increased recovery, higher tolerance to lactic acid, increased VO2 Max	Anatomical Adaptation	Increase in Anaerobic Threshold, increased anaerobic enzymes for more efficient use of fat as a fuel source at higher intensities, heart rate efficiency

Intervals like the example above are great because they allow for greater efforts over a shorter period of time. Don't be fooled, however – intervals can be done lower levels of intensity too – and in any sports that you cross train in (swimming, cycling, inline skating, etc.)

Functions of Training - prescriptions for training in terms of frequency, intensity, time and measurements for each.

Functions of Training for Triathlon Running

Triathlon running is a tough method to learn. Even very quick athletes with solid distance running backgrounds are dumbfounded initially by the adjustment required to run after swimming and cycling. Beginner runners who are intimidated by the idea of even participating in a triathlon are often times put at ease with the idea that the "run" can actually be a "walk", both in training AND in racing. There is no rule that says a runner has to run the race and most certainly anyone wanting to merely finish the race, which is a victory in itself, can always hold tight to this security blanket.

Walking is a form of running many elite runners become aware of too, most often after a day of hard racing when proper training or nutrition was for one reason or another not part of their race mix. A very high percentage of Ironman triathletes end up walking in their races. There is no shame in finishing, but everyone will admit that it is a little more fun (and sometimes gratifying to the ego) when you can finish with flair.

The following are example workouts for three weeks of triathlon running. Again, these workouts reiterate the 9 key workout principle, providing three major cycling workouts per week in the following three categories of training:

* Intervals
* Long Workout
* Threshold Workout

Any of the following workouts can be modified for various distances. It is also important to note that these workouts are not written in a progression based model, meaning that they are example workouts from various weeks during the training season and don't represent the first three weeks in a row of training. The purpose of these workouts are to give you an overview of some types of workouts both advanced and beginners alike can modify to fit their talents, goals, and needs.

For a tailored training plan for you, please email: shawnboom@attbi.com.

Week #1 Running Workouts

Intervals

Warm Up

5K – 1/2 marathon runners: 12 x 400 meters @ 90-93% MHR for advanced / 80-90% for beginners

Long course triathletes: 5 x 6 minutes at 87-90% MHR

Cool Down

Threshold Workout

"Anaerobic Threshold Test"

Warm Up to your comfort level

2 x 20 minutes as hard as you can go (active rest between intervals)

Cool down

The average of your heart rates for the first 20 minutes and the second 20 minutes, averaged together is your approximate anaerobic threshold heart rate. For example, if I averaged 180 beats in the first 20 minutes and 190 beats in the second, my estimated anaerobic threshold heart rate would be
(180 + 190) / 2 = 185

Long Run

1 hr. 15 min @ 75-85% MHR. The goal here being to maintain a steady heart rate throughout the entire long run. Experienced athletes and beginners alike should stick to the time provided and put their mental efforts into holding as steady a heart rate as possible.

Week #2 Running Workouts

Intervals

Note: Do this workout in the Power phase of training.

> 6 x 2 minute hills
>
> Find a hill that takes about 2 minutes. Run up it at 87% and recover back down to 60%. Repeat 6 times. Warm up and cool down 15 minutes each.

Threshold Workout

> 20 minute warm up.
>
> 4 x 5 minutes at your anaerobic threshold +3 beats
>
> Cool down 25 min.

Long Run

> 2 hr 30 minutes @ 5-8 Beats below AT running AT

Test your race pace of 5—8 beats lower than AT for long course. Short course triathletes should cut the time down to 2 hours and concentrate on their race pace being around (or above AT) which means the long run shouldn't be run at race pace.

Week #3 Running Workouts

Intervals

20 Min warm up

15 min @ 88%

8 min @ 64%

10 min @ 89%

8 min @ 63 %

5 min @ 90%

Cool down 5 min @ 60 %

Threshold Workout

9 Miles (beginners, cut this distance to 6 miles total)

Warm Up 20 min.

Do 8 x 5 minutes @AT +3.

Recover 3 minutes at 60% between intervals.

Focus on building strength and endurance in the intervals.

Cool Down 10 + min

Long Run

3 hours @ AT pace minus 5 beats. Test this pace and heart rate and see how it feels. If you are unable to sustain the pace, drop another 5 beats. Decide what heart rate you want to race your triathlon at. Olympic distance triathletes should cut this workout to 2 hours in length and aim for a pace of AT minus 3 beats.

Running Key Workouts

Run Key Workout #1 - 20, 15, 10, 5 Run Workout

The greatest way to improve your endurance is doing interval workouts that make you recover at a high percentage of your max heart rate. This one should be done anytime during your periodization cycle after your base phase is complete. You have to know your AT before doing this workout.

20 Minutes warm up @ 75% MHR

20 Minutes @ AT heart rate

5 Minutes @ 75% MHR (active recovery)

15 Minutes @ AT heart rate

5 Minutes @ 75% MHR (active recovery)

10 Minutes @ AT heart rate

5 Minutes @ 75% MHR (active recovery)

5 Minutes @ AT heart rate

5 Minutes @ 65% MHR cool down

Run Key Workout #2 - Mile Repeats Running

Building Speed is essential to race preparation if competing is your goal. If you are not feeling the competitive urge for a race, it is not necessary to complete workouts like this one. If you want to be ahead of the field, you CANNOT skimp or miss these intervals. They are simple, time tested, and essential to your program! You'll notice that in the mile intervals, you can choose between 3 to 8 repetitions. It is a good idea to start with 3 and add one or two each week until you reach the number 8. This type of a workout should be done in the 2 months prior to your race.

15 minute warm up @ 70% MHR

3 – 8 x 1 mile @ 90-95% MHR with ? the time it took you to finish the last mile as your recovery at 65% MHR.

10 minute cool-down @ 70% MHR

Equipment and Tips

Overhauling the gear closet, what is necessary, what is luxury, what is ludicrous. Running is an eloquently simple sport. The equipment needed is pure and the benefits are astounding. Like anyone driving an old car, however, runners like to dream of the gear that'll "get em there" faster.

Essentials

- Shoes
- Socks
- Carry-along Water Bottle
- Sunscreen
- Hat
- Sun Glasses
- Running Shorts (or Speedo with regular shorts)

Luxury

- Heart Rate Monitor
- Speed / Distance Monitor
- Racing Flats
- Head phones
- More time to run than a 1 hour lunch hour
- Personal Coach
- Training Partner

Ludicrous

- Skinny body

CHAPTER 6

The JULSTRO™ Method of Self-treatment

The Julstro Technique is a deep muscle therapy that grew out of years of treating clients, many of them athletes, with various musculoskeletal injuries. When athletes train they spend hours doing strength movements, contracting the muscles to lift weights, swim, run, cycle, etc. The muscles become overused, and the athlete now has a "repetitive strain injury" that prevents him/her from moving the strained area without pain.

Deep muscle therapy would stop the pain, but the athlete would return to the previous level of exercise, and the problem would come back. I needed to develop a self-treatment system, so that athletes could stop the pain completely, by themselves!

This book will instruct you how to properly self-treat each muscle spasm or contraction. You will become so comfortable with the Julstro Self-Treatments, that you will find your hand automatically going to the correct area whenever you feel a pain in the joint, or in the muscle itself.

While I wouldn't have thought it at the time, I had the "good fortune" of having a lot of painful conditions stop me in my tracks. I didn't know any therapist who could do what I knew needed to be done, so I began to treat myself – and this was the beginning of the Julstro Self-Treatment System. I found that if I could work out a treatment on myself, I could easily teach a client to do the same.

Eventually, as the various methods were developed, I found that teaching my patients how to do the techniques gave them the ability to continue their treatments at home, enhancing the benefits of their office sessions. Since I have joined my practice with Dr. Cohen, the Julstro techniques have been brought to a new level. Throughout this book I will use the pronoun "we" to designate the times when Dr. Cohen was involved. We work together as a team, each adding a piece of expertise that enhances the other, and you receive the benefit of both of us.

There are several advantages to deep muscle therapy: first and foremost, deep therapy brings fresh blood to the muscle, bringing nutrients to the muscle fibers. One of the by-products of muscle action is lactic acid, and when this builds up the muscle is denied access to fresh blood. Our body has a mechanism to release the lactic acid - if we give it enough time. However, modern life keeps us so busy that we keep creating lactic acid, not flushing it away. Working deeply on the muscle is like having a pump for the muscle - when you press down deeply you are pushing the lactic acid out; when you release, blood fills the void.

Deep muscle therapy also stretches the muscle fibers, and releases any contractions or spasms. This allows the joint to move more freely, giving you a better range-of-motion.

When doing the deep movements that are included in the Julstro Technique it is important not to let your fingers (or whatever is providing the pressure) slide on the skin. Did you ever have "rug-burn"? Sliding on the skin while doing deep muscle therapy can cause the skin to have that same feeling.

Prior to treatment, put heat onto the area. Chronic, tight muscles respond well to the comfortable warmth, which will eventually help to release the tightness, making it easier to treat and stretch the muscles.

We also advise people to use a deep-muscle cream, such as Sombra', to help the muscle fibers relax. Put a generous amount on the entire muscle and if possible, place a heating pad over it for 5 minutes prior to doing self-treatment or stretching. You will need to wait until the cream is completely absorbed before you can treat the muscle.

When a muscle is bruised use ice to stop the further bruising. Ice is beneficial when an injury has just occurred within the previous 24 hours. We suggest applying ice after doing any very deep therapy to a muscle. Occasionally deep therapy will bruise fibers, and the day after treatment you may feel like you bumped into a piece of furniture – this is temporary. You may even occasionally see a bruise on your skin. This is not serious, and is no reason for concern, any discomfort goes away in 24-48 hours, and on the plus side, you'll already be moving more easily. When using an ice compress, never put the ice directly on your skin, and never leave it on for more than fifteen minutes at a time. We have also found that arnica gel, which is available at any health food store, is great for healing bruised muscles.

When doing deep muscle therapy we suggest you work each area to your tolerance level. Try to reach for the "hurts so good" level – you'll know it when you reach it! If you don't go deeply enough, you are only treating the surface muscles. You need to apply sufficient pressure to reach the deep muscles. Drink a lot of water after each treatment to help flush away toxins that have been released into your system.

How to Work on Your Own Muscle Spasms

Trigger Points: Spasms, Contractions and Adhesions

The following information will help you learn how to "feel" a trigger point.

Spasms are also known as "trigger points"; the terms will be used interchangeably throughout the book. A spasm of the muscle fibers causes pain, or discomfort, in the muscle or the joint that it is moving.
It is easy to learn how to work on your own muscle spasms. The first thing is to learn how to feel the difference between a spasm, a contraction, and an adhesion.

Healthy muscle feels firm but flexible. Depending on its size it will have hundreds or thousands of fibers lying next to each other in nice straight lines.

Spasms and Trigger Points

A spasm, or Trigger Point, is a knot of muscle fibers that feels like a hard bump in the muscle, like a frozen pea.

To work on a spasm, center your finger - or other source of pressure such as a tennis ball, a dowel, or a rolling pin - directly on top of the spasm, push straight down, pressing for about 30 seconds, and then move an inch or so in either direction. Repeat the treatment. Do this several times in different areas immediately surrounding the spasm. As long as you are not sliding on the skin, you will be doing just fine. Here's a hint; if you find you can't easily glide from one treatment area to the next area, put powder on your hands and rub it in - using oil is not as effective as powder because you will keep slipping as you work deeply on the muscle.

Contractions

A contraction is a shortening of the muscle, and depending on its size or location it feels like a thick rope within the muscle, or the entire muscle may feel thick and hard. To visualize a contraction, think of taking the muscle and pushing the two ends into the center, making the muscle shorter and thicker. The problem is, in our bodies each of the two ends of the muscle is still connected to a bone - and the shortening causes a great deal of tension on the bones. In fact, if the muscle contracts too much it will actually tear from the bone. This is the situation when a person has an Achilles tendon tear at the heel of the foot, shin splints, or a torn hamstring.

To work out a contraction, press down and hold for about 30 seconds, then press down and pull at the same time, going only to the end of the skin's elasticity. Don't slide on the skin. Do this several times. Pick up your fingers just a little, letting the skin release before you put your fingers down again to repeat the movement. This will all be clear as we go through each individual technique.

Another way of treating the muscle is, whenever possible, grip the entire contraction with your whole hand. We tell our clients to grab the muscle as if you were grasping a thick cucumber, and then squeeze it tightly. If you squeeze, and pull at the same time with the intention of lengthening the muscle, you will accomplish flushing and stretching the muscle in one movement.

Do each of these techniques along the entire length of the muscle. You will find that each time you do the movements it will hurt less. This is because the spasms and contractions are lengthening, and the tension is being released from the muscle fibers.

Adhesions

Adhesions are the body's way to protect an injured muscle fiber, and is actually a phenomenon called "splinting". If a fiber gets injured, the muscle puts out a sticky substance that causes the fibers next to the injured fiber to stick, allowing the injured fiber to relax because it is being carried along with the adjoining fibers. This reduces the power of your muscle by taking some of the fibers out of action. Instead of each fiber working independently, giving you the ability to use all the fibers required to do the task you want, the center fibers are not working at all, decreasing your strength.

Adhesions feel like tight strings. To break them down you go across them like you are playing a guitar. Adhesions aren't usually painful; in fact you rarely know they are there. Eventually you will begin to realize that you don't have the power that you once had, and you don't know why.

Having worked with thousands of clients, we have found that in many cases muscles are overlooked when physicians are diagnosing painful joint problems. This is particularly true of carpal tunnel syndrome and low back pain: the muscles in the area are rarely even considered before surgery is planned. Dr. Cohen and I both believe it behooves everyone, prior to having surgery on any joint, as well as back surgery, to first check the muscles that are affecting the joint. The best person to examine the muscle is a massage therapist who does deep tissue therapy, and is fully trained in muscles, their actions, referred pain areas, and the reaction of the body to contractions of the muscle.

While other types of therapies concentrate on ligaments, bones, and the nervous system, deep muscle therapy concentrates solely on the action of muscles on the joints. Massage therapists are trained to use the sensitivity of their hands to find and treat these problems.

Spasm Relief Tools – Tennis Balls and Clothes Poles!

When I began teaching our clients how to treat their own spasms I found that some people had difficulty because of lack of flexibility. In some cases, such as the back, the area couldn't be reached without the aid of a tool, and for other areas strength was a problem. As a result, several simple tools became the method of choice. In this book I'll be showing you how to do the treatments using your own hands and arms, and also using a variety of simple "tools" such as a length of 1" thick dowel (commonly used as a clothes pole in your closet), a door jam, a tennis ball, or a golf ball.

Anyone who purchases the Julstro Video System for the treatment of wrist/hand pain and numbness, commonly related to the symptoms of Carpal Tunnel Syndrome, will also receive a specially designed tool, called the Julstro Tool. This tool has many uses throughout the body. Proper use of the Julstro Tool for the forearm and hand is explained in the video package.

It has been fun working with each client to decide which tool will work best. As we worked closely with serious athletes who compete in 26.2 mile marathons, 100+ mile cycling races, and Ironman competitions, we have found how to do the Julstro Technique "on the run". Dr. Cohen and I appreciate your input - and are happy to be beneficial to you and to your sport!

When to Use Heat and Cold Packs

Dr. Cohen suggests that the rule of thumb is: cold if the injury is less than 24-36 hours old (called "acute"), and heat when the injury is of longer duration (called "chronic"). Also, if there is considerable pain, regardless of whether the injury is acute or chronic, the cold pack will help to numb the area and give relief.

After doing a strenuous exercise program, or after working deeply on a muscle, always use ice to heal any muscle trauma. Never put ice directly onto the skin, put cloth between the ice and the skin to prevent freezing of the skin tissue. Ice should only be applied for 15 minutes at a time. Let the skin return to body temperature for 15 minutes and then apply again if necessary. If the skin is cold for longer than 15 minutes at a time it can cause damage to the skin and muscles.

The body has an innate intelligence that will tell us whether to use heat or cold. If we imagine putting heat on an area, and then think how it feels, and do the same with imagining cold on the area, we will know our body's answer.

CHAPTER 7

The Trigger Point Charts

Finding the Source of Pain

In Chapter 1 Dr. Cohen explained muscle action and the term "Trigger Point". This book uses colorful trigger point charts, which were drawn by Jerry Trump from the research published by Janet Travell, MD, and David Simon, MD. The charts will to help you find the source of your pain.

The abbreviation "TP" will be used to designate the Trigger Point Charts. The abbreviation "M" will be used to designate the Muscle Charts which have been included for your convenience.

On the TP charts you will see circled "x" marks; these are the trigger points. You will also see areas shaded in the same color. The darker colored area is the primary point of referred pain, and the lighter shaded areas may be involved to a lesser degree. The name of the muscle is printed in the same color as its corresponding area of pain.

When you locate the area where you are feeling pain on the chart, go to the name of the muscle in the caption under the index to find where the treatment for that muscle is located.

An important fact is that the "x" may be so far away from the referred pain area that it is actually on two different figures on the chart! Also, an "x" may be shown on the left, or right, side of the body. We have the same muscles on both sides of our body, and the spasm could be on either side. The chart shows it on only one side so as not to have to be repeated.

The body is extremely predictable. Pain "refers" (is felt) in areas distant from the trigger point: for example, notice on TP Chart 1 that a trigger point in the neck has a pain referral in the chest, the upper back, the entire length of the arm and the hand! This caused us a moment's uncertainty about where we should put the treatment for a trigger point in the neck: should it go in the chest, back, arm, or hand? We decided to always put the treatment in the section where the pain would be felt.

As more and more athletes came to us with sports-related injuries, either through online forums or in the office, we worked together to develop ways for them to do the self-treatments during their training sessions - and even during a competition.

The Muscle Charts have been included to help you understand the text regarding each muscle. You will see the origination and insertion of each muscle, and you will be able to clearly understand how the muscle can cause pain far from the site of the spasm.

One last thought. Muscles have long, and sometimes complicated, Latin names. While it is not necessary for you to learn the names of the muscles, we will use them so you will be able to locate the trigger points on the charts.

PART III
THE JULSTRO TREATMENTS

CHAPTER 8

The Core of the Body

The Iliopsoas:

The Foundation of the Body and Source of Multiple Problems!

It is amazing to learn that one muscle group, the Iliopsoas, commonly called the psoas (pronounced "so-as") can cause pain from the head to the toes. But it is absolutely true! We guarantee that most medical doctors, or therapists, will not consider your psoas muscle when you present to their office with joint pain or numbness anyplace in the body.

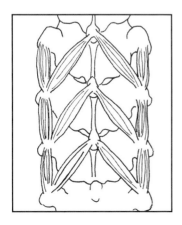

Before we examine the psoas, let's look at the logic behind the muscles that move the spine, and how the psoas causes such a wide area of pain.

Each vertebre of your spinal column sits on top of another vertebre. From your head to your sacrum, each vertebre is connected by small muscles called multifidi. As demonstrated in the graphic to the left, each multifidus muscle connects the vertebre on top to the one just below it.

There is also a long muscle called Erector Spinae that begins at the skull and ends at the sacrum area. While it appears to be one long muscle, it is actually thousands of individual fibers that originate on your ribs and insert onto the vertebre sometimes several levels higher or lower.

As each of these muscle fibers contract, the vertebre moves in that direction. It is an amazing system that allows us to bend our backs in the wide variety of movements that we take for granted – until something goes wrong!

The psoas muscle is the most incredible of these muscles because it connects the upper body to the lower body, and spasms anyplace along the length of the muscle will cause the vertebre of the low back to compress, and will also cause the vertebre of the upper/mid back to change alignment, referring pain into that area.

The Lower Back

> **Since there could be complicating issues, it is suggested that you visit your physician if you have been having lower back pain.**

Pain in the low back is something that at least 70% of our clients complain about. And it is one of the most misunderstood conditions. The muscles involved are the erector spinae, and the iliopsoas, which is called simply the psoas (pronounced "so-as").

It will help if you take a look at M Chart 8 – psoas, and M Chart 10 – erector spinae, while you are reading this explanation.

The erector spinae muscles are a large grouping of three separate muscles all closely placed together. Some originate on the ribs, others originate on the entire length of the spine, on each vertebra, they cause us to stand up from a bent position, and to be able to twist and turn our trunk.

The psoas originates on the lumbar (low back) vertebrae, it goes forward (behind your intestines), goes inside the bowl of your hips, and then inserts into the front of the femur (thigh bone).

The psoas muscle pulls you down, so you can touch the floor, and the erector spinae pull you back up to the standing position.

The psoas is also instrumental in lifting your leg to take a step, or pedal a bike.

Let's spend a few minutes describing the location and action of each of these muscles. Cross your arms so your hands are back-to-back, with your fingers touching and pointing at the ceiling. Your left hand (which is now on your right) will be erector spinae, and your right hand (which is now on your left) will be psoas.

When you bend, for example; to ride a bike or to touch the floor, the psoas contracts and you are pulled over. Try it with your hands to demonstrate. Keep the back of the hands together and fold your right fingers down toward your palm. You can imagine the opposing muscle (erector spinae) needing to stretch to be able to do this move. When you stand back up straight, erector spinae contracts and psoas needs to relax. To demonstrate that movement pull the fingers of your left hand up straight, and have your right hand follow.

The problem comes from the fact that with every step, and each time we sit down, the psoas contracts. We do this many thousands of times every day, and unless we fold over backward, it never gets stretched! Both of these muscles originate on the lumbar vertebrae (low back), when either one of them goes into a spasm they pull on the vertebrae, and the pain is felt in the low back.

Since the erector spinae is stretching many thousands of times every day, it rarely goes into a spasm in the low back area – but it is common for the psoas to become contracted because of the phenomenon called "muscle memory". As the muscle contracts in a spasm it pulls the lumbar vertebrae forward and down, and you feel the pain in your low back. People automatically rub their back, but the pain is actually coming from the muscle that is located on front of the spine, and behind your intestines.

This is the reason why the pain actually feels a bit better when you bend over – you are going into the contraction and taking the pressure off the lumbar vertebrae. But, when you stand up, the muscle is again pulling on the vertebrae: pulling the bone out of alignment; compressing the disks; impinging on the nerves; and you are also feeling the tug of the muscle on the bone. If the psoas is severely contracted it becomes difficult to bend your leg, and even just picking your foot up off the floor is a problem. The muscle definitely needs to be stretched!

While working with athletes who come to our forum (www.julstro.com) we have found that a contracted psoas will rotate the pelvis forward and down, and therefore cause the hip muscles to all become torqued and therefore will pull improperly:

The twisted tensor fascia lata on the lateral side of the hip (and therefore the iliotibial band – ITB) will cause pain to be felt in the knee, and will cause a misalignment that will effect the lower leg all the way down to the ankle.

The rotated pelvis will cause the hamstrings to become overstretched, with pain felt in the buttocks and posterior knee. The muscle will also appear to be in contraction because it is very tight, making the athlete believe he/she needs to stretch the fibers. This will complicate the problem and can cause severe muscle tearing.

The rotated pelvis will press up onto the sciatic nerve, and it can overstretch the piriformis muscle.

The overstretched piriformis muscle will press down onto the sciatic nerve, referring pain across the buttocks, into the hip, down the posterior leg and into the foot.

The quadriceps go into spasm creating a strain on the insertion point below the kneecap.

The most dramatic example of the result of pain in the psoas muscle that we have ever seen came from a new client named Leon. He had suffered from pain in his low back for two years, sought various treatments from a wide variety of therapists, and ultimately had surgery on his low back. After surgery, the pain stayed at exactly the same intensity, and in the same place! He then spent months in physical therapy, and still the pain remained. He had enjoyed running and playing tennis prior to this painful condition, and that was no longer a part of his life.

Then he started getting pain in his thigh and again went to the doctor, who told him it was scar tissue that had wrapped around his nerve, and it needed to be surgically removed. He said "no" and

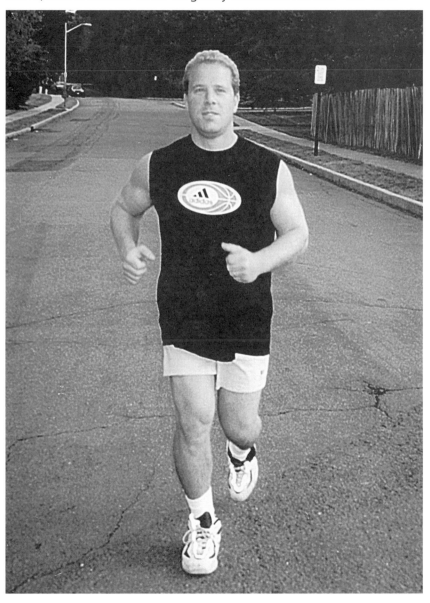

came to see us. When he described the pain, I immediately thought of the psoas muscle, and sure enough, when I touched it Leon yelped in pain. The treatment was painful, but we worked together to keep it well within his pain tolerance level, and at the end of the treatment he said his back felt "80 % better."The next week the contraction released the other 20% and his low back pain stopped completely. Leon returned to his physician, who was shocked at the result. Unfortunately, this physician did not decide to learn why the psoas was involved, or how he could check for contractions in the psoas muscle in order to prevent this from happening to future patients.

"After living in pain for over a year, and subsequently having unsuccessful back surgery, I was told I'd never run again. Fortunately I met Julie and learned a few simple stretches and techniques, and I'm back on the road. These techniques really work – try them – you have nothing to lose but your pain!" Leon

The second piece to this story, that discusses the pain in the front of Leon's thigh, is in the chapter about the upper leg.

We have worked with hundreds of clients who have been relieved of their chronic pain in various parts of their bodies, and as long as you are cleared medically, we believe that this stretch for the low back can also help you.

As mentioned, the psoas never gets stretched. There are three ways of doing this effectively; you can use whichever way feels best for you. Remember to only go to the point of a " feel good" stretch, not to the point of causing sharp pain. You will be able to go further each time you do it, and your back will feel better each time. As soon as you feel the stretch, slowly stand up straight. Don't hold yourself in the painful position. You'll be amazed at how quickly this helps low back pain!

Turn around at the sink – putting your calves up against the cabinet, and your hips resting against the counter. Keep your hips and calves touching the cabinet, also keep facing straight ahead, and lean back, moving your upper back over the sink. It helps if your lift up your chest, like you are trying to make a backward arch with your chest. This will raise the spine a bit before you lean back. Do this movement 10 times. On the last stretch bend forward, arching your back and moving your hips side to side.

Another method is done by lying on the floor on your stomach.

Do a modified push-up keeping your hips firmly on the floor, and bending backward at the waist. Go only until you feel a comfortable stretch, hold it for 6 seconds, and then come back flat onto the floor again.

Do this 10 times, trying to stretch a bit further each time.

On the last stretch, finish by folding at the hips and sitting on your feet. Stretch your back and put your head on the floor.

Finally, after you have stretched the psoas, it is important to treat the insertion point at the front of your thigh, and also to treat the quadriceps muscle (see – The Upper Leg). We have never had a client with psoas contractions who didn't also have a big spasm in the lateral (outside) portion of their quadriceps muscle.

Sit down and find the crease where your hip meets your leg. Then go to the center of the crease.

Put your elbow directly onto the crease. Add pressure by pressing down with your shoulder. You'll know when you are near the spot. Hold the pressure for 60 seconds without pain. Continue doing the treatment until you feel the pain lessening.

You want to feel the pressure deep into the muscle and hip joint, while still staying in the tolerable range.

To stretch this area go to the section on quadriceps.

This is one of the "dual purpose treatments". As you are treating the insertion point of the psoas, you are also treating the origination of the quadriceps – and relieving pain in the anterior portion of your hip! This is a good time to continue the treatment and go down the entire quadriceps muscle.

The Quadratus Lumborum

The Quadratus Lumborum, "QL" for short, is the muscle that most people rub when they have low back pain. However, in our clinical practice we've found that it isn't the primary cause of low back pain - the psoas holds that distinction.

The action of the QL is to pull you over to the side, and it also picks up your hip so you can make a step – or sit down. Every time you pick up your foot the QL is contracting to allow that movement, and every time you sit down it is contracting to enable you to bend your leg. You can see how it can easily become overworked.

Notice that the referred pain for the QL, shown on TP Chart 11, is the same as that for the psoas. This is because, when you are sitting for a long period of time, or you have been running, walking or climbing stairs, the muscle has contracted. Then you try to stand up straight, but the muscle is too short for you to do that, so it pulls the lumbar vertebrae out sideways. This puts severe pressure on the spinal cord at the lumbar region, and you have low back pain!

Any sport that requires a great deal of running: soccer players; football and basketball players; tennis; and naturally, runners, have a propensity for spasms in the QL muscle. Because of the location of the pain, you rub your low back. However, the muscle is underneath the very strong muscle of the back – the Erector Spinae. To effectively treat this muscle you need to stretch the fibers fully.

The stretch for the QL muscle is very effective, and one that has you looking like a pretzel.

Put your hand on your low back, at the curve of your waist, you'll be right on the QL. Since the muscle goes up and down between the last of your ribs and your hips, the only way to stretch it is to move those two points apart. By adding a little bit of a twist to the movement, you get a better stretch than by just bending over to the side.

Stand up with your butt pressed up against a wall. For demonstration purposes we'll stretch the right side, so you'll be bending to the left.

Keeping your butt on the wall, lean over to the left and then twist to try to touch your right hand to the back of your left leg. You won't be able to do it; in fact, you won't even be able to get close to the back of your leg. Just try to go as far as you can without moving your butt away from the wall.

Move your body about until you find the best stretch in your low back. Naturally, do this same stretch on the opposite side, even if you aren't having any pain in that area. The body compensates when we are in pain and we frequently will be straining the opposite muscle.

Again, be sure to keep this stretch at the "feels good" level.

CHAPTER 9

The Many Faces of Hip Pain

The hip is second only to the shoulder in the amount of flexibility that it allows, and yet we pay little attention to its mobility…until something goes wrong!

Our hips swivel in an amazing number of angles, each movement being directed by a separate set of muscles all working in unison. Remember, muscles are like a pulley system. For any movement to happen, one set of muscles must contract, while the opposing set of muscles must relax. As a result, the potential for any one of those muscles going into spasm, and altering the function of all the other muscles, is enormous!

Athletes have a disproportionate amount of hip pain because of the frequency and duration of exercise periods. Many sports such as: cycling, running, bodybuilding, tennis and golf, etc., place an enormous amount of stress on the hip muscles. The fact that these are all done repetitively in the exact same direction causes specific muscles to spasm, with common areas of pain developing for each sport.

Fortunately the muscles are all close together, so treating one muscle usually benefits several other muscles. We will be addressing the major muscles in each area, but you are actually working on many muscles with each treatment.

This chapter and the shoulder chapter compete as potentially the longest in the book – there are so many spasms that cause hip & shoulder pain. You will be using a tennis ball frequently for the deep muscle treatments. Roll onto the ball slowly, and always stop before the pain passes your tolerance level. With that in mind, let's begin with the #1 cause of hip pain: piriformis syndrome, which often causes the pain of sciatica.

Sciatica – A Real Pain in the Butt!

The interesting thing about sciatica pain (if there can be an interesting thing about pain!) is that you cannot find a position that relieves the pain, and yet a simple stretch can alleviate it totally.

The sciatic nerve is actually the continuation of the spinal cord. When the cord reaches the sacrum (the flat bone at the base of your spine) it splits in two. Each division is now called the sciatic nerve. The sciatic nerve travels through an opening in the pelvis, and down the back of the leg. The complicating factor here is that the piriformis muscle originates at exactly the same point where the sciatic nerve exits the pelvis, through an area called the Greater Sciatic Notch. When the muscle goes into a spasm it presses the sciatic nerve into the bone - causing the symptoms of sciatica.

The piriformis muscle is frequently overlooked completely, and yet when one thinks of the anatomical placement of the muscle and nerve, it is the first thing that should be addressed when evaluating sciatica.

Actually, a better name for the pain you are experiencing is Piriformis Syndrome.

Charlie Chaplin's famous walk is an example of severe piriformis contraction. People who are most prone to piriformis syndrome are: runners, people who climb many stairs or work out on a stair climbing machine, individuals who sit for many hours at a time (including in a car or at a desk), and men who keep their wallets in their back pockets.

Several years ago we had a client who had an extreme case of Piriformis Syndrome. Jan was only 27 years old when she developed hip pain. The pain kept her up at night, and was with her all day. Her doctor ordered x-rays, and an MRI. Everything came back negative.

Eventually she was sent for physical therapy, but to no avail. The pain continued to get worse. After several YEARS of pain she was referred to a psychiatrist, who told her it was "all in her head" and put her on Prozac. Meanwhile, all of her friends were having fun, skiing, dancing, meeting men, and getting married – Jan was almost crippled from the pain and could not go out. She was depressed, and ate candy, not carrots. Needless to say, she gained lots of weight. This not only lowered her self-esteem, it increased her pain. Complicating her life further was the fact that she was in a dead-end job because it allowed her unlimited sick time.

When we first met Jan, she had been suffering for seven years. She walked with a cane and was bent over at the waist. Jan walked on her right toes because she could no longer straighten her leg. Her head was arched up to compensate for the bend in her back. Ironically, she came to the Julstro Center for shoulder pain. When asked why she was walking the way she was, she told us her story.

We thought, "With all the professionals who have seen this lady in the past seven years, it can't be just Piriformis Syndrome. Surely, one of them would have looked at the piriformis." Yet, Jan told us that no one had ever touched the muscle, they just gave her exercises, or pain medications.

Simply touching her piriformis muscle caused her to scream. It was so contracted that it felt like a bone! I began working with her, very gently at first, in order to bring some blood into the area, and soften the muscle.

After the first hour's treatment, Jan stood up. She was still bent over, and still stood on her toe. When I asked her if she was in pain, she said "no", so I told her to slowly put her foot on the floor – stopping when she felt pain. Miraculously, she was able to put her foot down flat on the floor. Then I told her to slowly stand up. Jan looked like a scared rabbit, and when she got all the way up straight, we both cried and hugged.

It took three months of frequent treatments, but one day Jan said "Julie, I can honestly say I have no pain in any part of my body!" We were thrilled. Unbelievably, her insurance wouldn't pay for deep muscle treatment, even though it paid for years of physical therapy, several MRI's, a psychiatrist, lots of Prozac, and many orthopedist appointments. Amazing!! This was one of the motivating factors for the development of the Julstro self-treatment system.

The location of the piriformis muscle is right under the hip pocket of your pants.

The piriformis originates on the sacrum (the big triangular bone at the base of your spine) and goes over to the hip (called the greater trocanter). The action of the piriformis is to turn your foot out.

The best way to self-treat the piriformis is to use a tennis ball. Lie on your back on the floor. If you are unable to lie on the floor, use a firm mattress. Have your knees bent and your feet flat on the floor.

Place the tennis ball where your back pocket would be, and GENTLY roll onto the ball. Keep within your pain tolerance level. Stay there for 30 seconds, and then roll further onto the ball. Do this until you are completely on the ball and you are feeling absolutely no pain. Then stay there for one full minute. If you feel pain during that minute, move off a bit, take a breath, and begin again. You should be able to stay on the ball for one minute comfortably.

Several years ago I had a personal bout with sciatica pain that ended up having me learn the best stretch I've ever encountered for the piriformis. I was told to do it every hour for several days, and while that may sound like a lot, it takes time for a muscle memory to change, and the muscle to attain a new, longer set point. This wonderful stretch has worked for me, and it's worked for many of our clients. It's easy to do, and the results are amazing!

The Piriformis Stretch

Stretching the piriformis muscle is the most beneficial treatment you can do to either prevent, or heal, the pain of sciatica. It's an easy stretch that is quick acting, if you do it properly, and frequently.

The key here is the placement of your knee as you move your leg. I think it's best to read this treatment and look at the pictures, then print out this page so you can look at the pictures again while you're actually doing the stretch.

Lie on your back, on the floor if possible, and bend both of your knees. You'll have the best results if you do this to both legs, even though you are only feeling the discomfort on one side of your body.

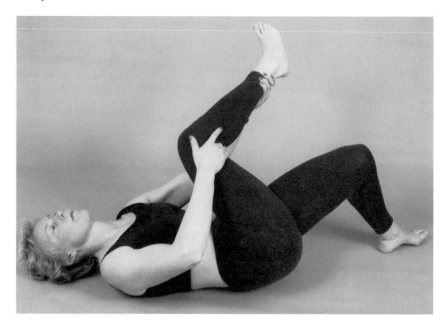

For demonstration purposes I'll show you how to stretch out your right muscle.

Bring your right knee to at least the middle of your body, having your knee in line with your nose. If you are flexible enough you can go further to the left, but you need to be at least at the midline.

If you find this position difficult, then this is your first goal to achieve. Once you have your knee at least at midline, hold it there with your right hand.

Next, put your left hand under your right ankle, and pull your right ankle up toward your left shoulder. Obviously you can't actually bring it there, just move it horizontally in that direction. Your level of flexibility will direct you regarding how far you can move.

Throughout this entire stretch, keep your back and shoulders flat on the floor.

For those less flexible, have someone help you with the stretch. Lie down, and while your assistant supports the weight of your leg with one hand, he/she guides your knee into midline. Once there, the assistant can begin to gently turn your leg to get the maximum stretch for the piriformis muscle.

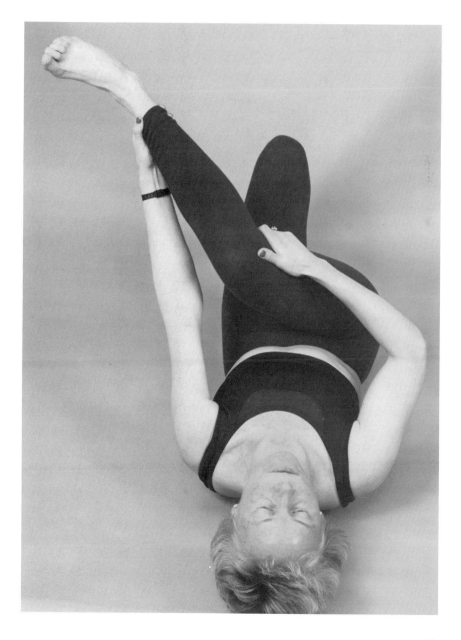

You'll feel a nice stretch in the buttock – the piriformis muscle. Keep the stretch at a level where it feels good – if it feels "sharp" back off a bit. The stretch needs to be held for one full minute. When the muscle feels like it's easing up, simply move your right foot more toward the left shoulder. Muscles need to be retrained to stay lengthened after they have been contracted for an extended length of time. The more times you do this stretch throughout the day, the faster the pain of sciatica will disappear. When we have a client who has a private office, we tell him/her to do it every hour! It works 95% of the time.

"It is amazing to me that we can treat ourselves!"

I first met Julie Donnelly at Ironman USA in Lake Placid. At the time I had a chronic ankle sprain and iliotibial band irritation from a previous marathon. She showed me in 10 minutes how to self treat my injuries. I was so impressed with my relief from the pain and the return to normal function that I subsequently signed up for her newsletter and have been consistently using her treatment system to treat any of my tight/overused muscles.

Annalisa

Age group triathlete, equestrian, and distance runner from Quebec Canada

The Gluteus Minimus –
The Second Most Common Source of Hip Pain

"After running hard, for over 2 hours, I had severe pain in my knee. I've already had personal experience using the Julstro techniques to heal several serious conditions, so I've come to know not to rub the area, but to look for the source of the pain. The pain was so severe I could barely walk, but the chart showed the spasm was in my hip, in the gluteus minimus, even though I didn't have any hip pain. When I pressed on the point that was shown in the chart, a searing pain shot down to my knee! I did the Julstro technique, alternating with the stretch, for 15 minutes. When I finished the pain was completely gone! I'm back to training at my optimal level, and I've added another preventative self-treatment to my routine." Jerry Trump

The gluteus minimus muscle and the tensor fascia lata are both responsible for pain in the knee, and for hip pain. The gluteus minimus also mimics the pain of sciatica. Look at Chart 14 and Chart 17 to see the referred pain areas from these two muscles; they cover a large percentage of your hip and leg!

The tensor fascia lata (TFL) muscle is right where your fists would go if you were putting them on your hips. The gluteus minimus muscle is at a point that is between the tensor fascia lata and the piriformis. The action of this muscle is to pull your leg directly out from the body. As a result, this is a muscle that is frequently strained in kickboxing, soccer, & wrestling, although it is a common area of pain for many people. The gluteus minimus is a major source of pain mimicking the same symptoms as the piriformis, and like the piriformis, the best self-treatment is with a tennis ball.

To find the proper place, stand up and feel your hips. Find the bone that is just below your waist, and then a few inches below it is the bone of your leg. The fleshy part in the middle is the gluteus minimus. Just below this spot is the tensor fascia lata muscle commonly called TFL.

Because the TFL muscle goes into a tendon that stretches all the way down to your knee, it refers pain to your knee. Most people don't think of their hips when the pain is at the knee!

The location of the piriformis is shown with an "x" (only shown on one side of the body). The tensor fascia lata is shown with arrows. The gluteus minimis is between the piriformis and the tensor fascia lata.

Working in this area, and moving the tennis ball just a little by just turning your body slightly, will get each of the muscles at the same time – it's one of the bonus treatments!

These muscles not only cause hip pain, but pain down the back of your leg (TP Charts 13, 14, and 17). You can alleviate lots of problems by working in this one area.

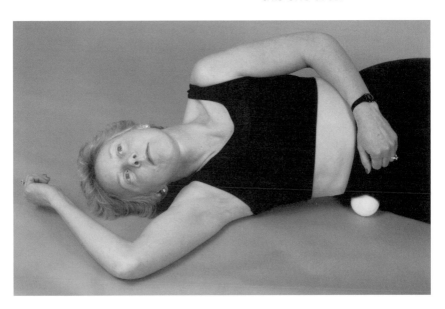

Now that you've found all of the muscles, lie down on your side. In order to treat the tensor fascia lata, put the tennis ball right at the fleshy part of the hip, and roll GENTLY onto the ball.

As always, stop if the pain starts moving toward intolerable. Hold each point for 60 seconds.

You will know instinctually when you are on the trigger point. It will be tender, and you'll know that you've found the problem.

After you work the TFL muscle, roll over a little onto your back.

You'll now be on the gluteus minimus, gluteus maximus, and gluteus medius in the back. Plus, with just a little movement you can reach the insertion point of the quadratus Lumborum by placing the ball on the top of your posterior pelvis.

The gluteus muscles are just about where your pant back pocket begins, and very close to the piriformis.

The following stretch for the TFL is for people who are flexible – and have good range-of-motion in their hips.

To demonstrate treatment on the left side of your body, put your left leg across the front of your right leg. Bring your left arm up and over your head, and bend toward the right side.

To get the full benefit, move your hips about a bit, until you feel the stretch. You should feel it about 3 inches back from your hipbone, and along your left posterior ribcage.

You can alter this stretch by moving your raised arm in different directions. This will give an additional stretch to the latissimus dorsi (Lats).

Insertion Point of the Psoas – A Source of Hip & Low Back Pain

Another place that causes low back pain, and anterior hip pain, is the point where the psoas muscle and the quadriceps meet. This point is directly at the top, and a little toward the outside, of the thigh. When you work on the quadriceps muscles (see - The Upper Leg), you will also be treating this source of the pain, however, the insertion point of the psoas is easy to treat by using your elbow.

While seated, find the crease where your abdomen meets your leg. Then go to the center of the crease. It's a bit tricky, but if you press around with your elbow, you'll locate it.

With your elbow on the crease, add pressure by pressing down with your shoulder and moving your elbow slightly toward your knee. You'll know when you are near the spot.

The idea is to hold the pressure for 60 seconds without pain.

Work with the pictures; they will help you do the treatments correctly. These treatments have been instrumental to many people in relieving their chronic hip pain; we hope they will be of benefit to you.

The quadriceps also cause pain in your hip. Each treatment assists in releasing the other muscle contraction. As a result, it will help if you combine this treatment with the treatment for the quadriceps.

However, we've found the quads usually affect the knee, more than the hip, so we've put the description of how to work them in the chapter for the upper leg.

CHAPTER 10

The Upper Leg - Knee and Hip Pain!

Working with Ironman Triathletes has been incredibly rewarding, and has demonstrated how important it is to work on the muscles of the quadriceps (called "quads" for short), the hamstrings in the thigh, as well as the gastrocneimus ("gastroc") in the calf. These muscles are a major cause of knee pain – for very logical reasons, once you understand the logic of the body.

Knee pain is a common complaint among all athletes. For example, cycling keeps the knees bent for extended periods of time, which will contract the hamstrings; and the forceful movement of pushing down on the pedals causes the quadriceps muscles to powerfully contract. Both of these muscles cross over the knee joint, and when the muscle is shortened from a contraction, it places enormous strain on the knee. Each muscle will pull on the knee joint, moving the bones out of alignment.

When a client comes in with knee pain, the first place we check are the quadriceps muscles.

Quadriceps - The front of the thigh – and Knee Pain

Because they originate on the front of the pelvic bone, when the quads are tight they throw the pelvis out of alignment. Think about what would happen if your pants were attached to the front of your hips, and you pulled down hard on them – you'd feel the pressure in your hips.

Likewise, if your pants were attached to just below your knee and you pulled up hard, you'd feel the pressure on your knee.

The quads are a major source of hip and knee pain for many people. The result of contracted quads, including a very common spasm that occurs midway down your thigh, either directly in the center, or just to the outside of the centerline (see TP Chart 17) is that your knee is being pulled toward the tight muscle. Frequently this is thought to be a ligament problem, however by simply releasing the spasms and stretching the fibers of the quad muscles you can totally relieve the knee pain.

Several years ago a client showed us how vital the "quads" are in relieving knee pain. She worked on a computer all day, and played tennis in her free time. She complained about her back and shoulders regularly, but never spoke about her knees. One day she said she was going in for knee surgery, and that she would be missing her next week's appointment. She was upset because she didn't think she'd be able to play tennis for two months.

I checked the quads since tight muscles would complicate recovery. On examination there was a huge spasm right in the middle of her thigh. It was 3 inches by 4 inches in size.

Releasing her quads was initially very painful, but as the contraction went down it became more tolerable, and eventually did not hurt at all.

We were surprised when she came in the next week for her regular appointment; we had expected her to be recuperating from the operation. She told us that when she went home after her appointment, her knee felt fine. Then the next day, her knee still felt fine. Since her knee pain had completely disappeared she canceled the surgery!

The second client was even more dramatic. Leon, who was discussed in the section on low back pain, came in to the office after having had unsuccessful surgery on his low back. After working out the muscle in his back, which relieved his back pain, he mentioned that he was having severe pain in his left thigh and hip. Leon runs on a regular basis, is an avid tennis player, and was told he could never play again! He had been told that scar tissue from the surgery had wrapped around the nerve, and he would need additional surgery. He absolutely refused, saying "I didn't need the first surgery; I'm not going for the second one!"

On examination, there was a huge spasm on his left thigh. Releasing the spasm had an immediate result. Leon got up from the chair and his pain had completely disappeared! Before explaining the treatment, let me finish by telling you that Leon has been able to go back to running and plays tennis every week. He's thrilled, and now that he knows how to treat his own leg and low back, he can be confident that the problem will not return.

If you look at the quadriceps, you will notice that the tendons of the quadriceps join together, and become the patella (kneecap) tendon. The tendon crosses directly over the kneecap and inserts on the bump just below the kneecap. Since the kneecap is a moveable bone, when a quad spasm pulls up on the tendon, the kneecap moves with it.

Depending on which of the four quadriceps muscles is doing the pulling, that is the direction that the kneecap will go, pulling the knee out of alignment.

The treatment that works best is to use an 18" piece of clothes pole – yes, the kind you'll find in your closet! While seated, use the clothes pole (a 1" dowel) to slide over the quads. Use as much pressure as you can tolerate.

Go all the way from the hip to the knee.

You can also use a rolling pin, however, don't hold it on the handles and let it roll, instead, hold it on the solid center, and slide it over the muscles.

The quads are big, thick muscles, so it will usually take several passes before you will begin to feel relief. If you find a particularly painful spot, just press down on it. The natural tendency for people is to avoid pain the moment they feel it, while just the opposite is what is necessary to relieve the spasm.

Do not go over the kneecap; stop about 2-3" before you reach that point. If you feel an area that is especially tender, you have found a spasm. Hold the pole on the spasm for a few moments, applying as much pressure as you can tolerate. Eventually this area will not be tender on subsequent treatments.

An alternative is to use your forearm. The bone, which goes from the elbow to the wrist, is your "rolling pin" (it's actually your ulnar bone).

To achieve the best results your thumb should be facing up. Lean in with your shoulder to put enough pressure on your quads. Simply push all the way down your thigh.

Do this several times, and always stay within your tolerance level. Remember, these are thick and deep muscles, so light pressure will not do.

As they say in the Marines "no pain – no gain", but with all of the Julstro treatments the pain must stay within your tolerance level.

The Quadriceps Stretch

The quads are very powerful muscles, and are also very difficult to stretch. Most people are familiar with the stretch that has you stand on one leg, taking the opposite ankle in hand, pull the leg back. This is effective to a degree. The two primary shortcomings are (1) some people can't balance on one leg, and (2) a stretch needs to be held for one minute. Also, if a spasm already exists, the stretch isn't effective in dissolving it. So, do the treatment described above, and then stretch the muscle.

The quadriceps are tricky muscles to stretch. If you kneel on the floor, sitting on your feet, you'll be in a good position to do an effective stretch.

Simply lean your body back and you'll feel the stretch. Hold the stretch for 60 seconds.

If you are very flexible you can lean all the way back to achieve the maximum stretch.

This is a treatment that anyone who runs, climbs lots of stairs, or drives for long distances should do. Rarely do the muscles themselves hurt– they usually refer pain to other places. You'll be pleased when you see how this helps to make you feel more flexible in both the knee and hip area.

Hamstrings – The Back of the Thigh

In 2001, I decided to learn how to ski. While on vacation, I had a serious accident – completely severing the MC (medial collateral) Ligament on the inside of the knee, and slightly tearing my AC (anterior cruciate) Ligament, which is in the back of the knee. These ligaments are the strong fibers that hold the knee together. When any of the ligaments tear the knee loses some of its stability, depending upon which ligament is involved.

The muscles of my quadriceps and hamstrings had contracted into multiple spasms that tightened the, causing a great deal of pain, and instability, in my knee. My knee felt like it was going to collapse toward the inside, and I felt shaky walking, and going up and down stairs. I didn't think I'd ever be able to ski again – since even walking was "tricky".

Immediately after the accident I began self-treating what felt like hundreds of spasms in my quads and hamstrings. The pain was so severe that even touching my thigh hurt, but I knew it had to be done. As the pain began to lessen, I thought "how glad I am that I know these techniques" and was more determined than ever to teach them to others.

After Dr. Cohen examined my knee, and did an MRI, we decided to concentrate on strengthening the hamstrings in order to give support to the knee. To relieve the tension on the knee joint I would also self-treat all the spasms in the hamstrings and quadriceps.

Eventually I was able to increase my level of exercise, and also the level of self-treatment techniques to dissolve the spasms and stretch the muscles. Surgery was avoided, and my knee is back to normal. This experience was the catalyst for the self-treatments for both the quads and the hamstrings. Again, finding the answer on myself has been the most successful way to knowing how to teach others.

I went back to skiing in 2002, and skied my best ever! I was thrilled! My knee was completely healed by using the Julstro Techniques.

A very effective way to work out the hamstrings is to use a ball and work down three lines, following the muscle from the top to the bottom. For as especially tight, or tender, muscle use a tennis ball on a soft chair.

To get more pressure, you can use a tennis ball, or baseball, on a hard surface. Look at TP Charts 13 & 14 for the referred pain areas of the hamstrings.

Begin by putting the ball at the very top of your leg. Make 3 lines down the back of your thigh. Begin all the way up at the crease in your thigh, where your buttocks meet your hamstrings, and work down each line to just above your knee. Sit down on the chair, putting your weight onto the ball, and hold it for 30 seconds before moving to the next point. You are looking for that "good hurt" here, don't overdo it.

CAUTION: DO NOT press the ball into the back of your knee!

Finish off this treatment by stretching the hamstrings, and quads.

The Hamstrings Stretch

The hamstrings are tight on almost everyone we work on, especially athletes, and people who sit for hours at a time. For those of you who are physically able, the best hamstring stretch looks awkward, but works great.

Sit on the edge of a chair with your feet spread shoulder width apart. Bend over and put your hands FLAT on the floor between your feet. Keep your head bent up toward the ceiling as far as possible to prevent dizziness. Then – stand up!

Sounds easy – until you try it. You'll quickly find out how contracted your hamstrings are when you do this stretch!

Here's the key. As the muscle fibers stretch you can keep pushing your knees a little further back. Every 15-30 seconds lift your butt a bit more by pushing your knees back, and therefore stretching the hamstrings. Keep it up until you either straighten your legs completely, or you decide to sit down and take a rest. Try to continue this stretch until you are straight legged.

If the muscle is "burning", keep your hands on the floor, sit down for 10 seconds, and then stand up again. You will be surprised at how much further your legs will straighten.

The beauty of this stretch is since you are starting with bent knees you cannot hyper-extend the joint, the position of your back is better for your spine, and the chair is right there should you get dizzy. You'll be pleased when you see how much better your legs will feel.

Another contributing factor to many people with knee pain is a muscle all the way up in the hip. The Latin name is Tensor Fascia Lata, and is called "TFL" for short. The chapter on hips gives you the method to work out the spasms in this area.

Groin Pull

The searing pain of a groin pull can stop an athlete short. The most common muscle to cause a groin pull is the gracilis muscle. This muscle originates on the pubic bone, crosses the back of the knee joint, and inserts into the inside border of the tibia (lower leg). When this muscle contracts it assists in bending your knee, it also rotates your knee inward, as a result, pain can be felt in the groin, or in the knee.

To feel the muscle contracting, sit in a chair, place your fingers on the inside of your thigh, at the top of your leg near the pubic bone, and then pull your knees together. You will feel the origination of the muscle contract. If you kick your foot out while you are running, you are straining the contracted gracilis muscle. You are also straining it when you work with abductor equipment at the gym. To balance the muscles of the inner and outer thigh, it is important to treat spasms in the gracilis, as well as spasms in the quadriceps, sartorius and tensor fascia lata.

When the muscle is contracted, and shortened by spasms, it pulls on either the knee joint or the pubic bone. As a result, this muscle refers pain to the groin and is often responsible for male athletes having pain in the prostrate area, and female athletes having pain in the ovarian area. Your doctor may do a complete work up for this, ALWAYS take the tests, but while you are waiting for the results, do the following treatment.

Sports such as running and biking are particularly hard on this muscle because they involve bending the knees. This pulls the muscle to its longest length. However, if the muscle is shortened by a spasm you will feel the tension at the groin or the knee.

The treatment is easy. Get an 18" length of clothes pole (like in your clothes closet) and sit at the edge of a chair. Place the pole as far up on the top of your inside thigh as possible, and GENTLY press down toward your knee.

This can be very painful, so go slowly.

The majority of the spasms will be found closer to the top of the inside thigh, but may go all the way down to just before the knee joint. As you self-treat, don't press into the pubic bone. You can take your fingers and gently press on the two insertion points at the pubic bone and the inside knee.

We suggest you put ice on the muscle after you work it out; also, arnica gel is great for bruised muscles. Apply it frequently over the entire area.

CHAPTER 11

The Lower Leg

> WARNING: Many conditions require medical attention from a
> qualified physician. "Bumps" in the tissue of the lower leg in
> particular, can be signs of a serious medical condition. Swelling of the
> lower limbs can also be symptoms of serious conditions as well. Never
> apply pressure to varicose veins. Always see your doctor before using
> the Julstro techniques.

The Nemesis of Many... The Source of Ankle and Foot Pain...and Shin Splints!

Shin Splints

A common complaint from athletes who do a lot of running in their
sport: soccer, tennis, basketball, football, baseball, as well as
running and jogging, is shin splints. Deep, burning, pain radiates
down the entire front of the lower leg, often from the knee to the
ankle. The pain can eventually become so severe that you can't
point your toes, and even slow walking is extremely painful.

The problem comes from a severely contracted tibialis anterior
muscle. Look at the tibialis anterior muscle and you will see that it is
a long thick muscle that runs along the entire length of the
shinbone, and its tendon inserts into the top outer portion of the
foot.

When the muscle of the shin is in spasm you can feel the pain either
as shin splints, or as pain in the outside/top ankle, depending on the
degree of the contraction and the exact location of the spasm. Look
at TP Chart 15 to see the referred area of pain. Notice that the pain
goes all the way to the toes.

If you run your finger directly down the muscle, while at the same
time bringing the front of your foot up off the floor, you will feel
the muscle contracting. Follow the muscle all the way over the front
of your ankle, just a bit toward the inside, and you will feel the
tendon as it tightens. The muscle then goes across the top of your
foot, under the arch and inserts on the bottom of your foot. As a
result this muscle can also cause pain in the arch.

Since the muscle contracts every time you lift up the front of your foot, every step you take contracts the muscle. If you run, and don't finish off each step by pointing your toes, you are contracting it far more than you are stretching it. Ultimately muscle memory sets in, and it shortens. As we have discussed throughout this book, when that happens the muscle pulls on the tendon and you feel pain at the insertion.

Many people experience pain from this muscle, for example those who do a lot of walking or driving. Runners are especially prone to experiencing pain at both the origination along the shinbone

because the muscle is actually pulling along the length of the bone; the top of the foot where it bends at the ankle; and the bottom of the foot because of the insertion of this muscle. When the tibialis anterior is contracted you frequently get a burning type of pain, or it feels like you banged it very hard and have a deep bruise. Each time you push off from a step, you point your toes down and pull the heel up. If you are feeling pain on the inside top of your foot, it is because the muscle is tight, or shortened, and now you are stretching it slightly with every step you take.

You must flush out the spasms, lengthen the contracted fibers, bring fresh blood into the area, and stretch!

Walk a little and watch the action of your foot. As you take a step you point your toes up, contracting the tibialis anterior (A) and stretching the calf muscles (B).

Then as you push off from your toes, you are stretching the tibialis anterior (A) and contracting the calf muscles (B).

When any of the muscles are shortened the pulling will hurt at the insertion point. The fact that the tendon goes under a band at the ankle, and that the tight tendons rub on the band, is the reason why this muscle can cause pain on the top of the foot close to the ankle.

The treatment is the same for both shin splints and ankle pain, so we'll discuss both here. Shin splints are a common condition for any sport in which running is an important component, especially if it is sustained running for any period of time. The tibialis anterior muscle contracts so strongly that it actually begins to pull away from the bone!

This treatment is easy, but it can be quite painful. We recommend warming the area before you do any deep therapy. You can warm it by taking a hot bath, using moist heat compresses, or prior to exercising you can use the heel of your opposite foot and quickly rub up and down the muscle.

The Julstro self-treatment for this condition is to lie down on the bed or floor. Have your lower leg exposed, or you may be more comfortable wearing tight pants, and remove your socks.

Demonstrated on the right leg: Take the heel of your left foot and place it just to the outside of the shinbone, all the way up near the knee. Now, apply pressure by pressing down on your left heel and DEEPLY slide down the right leg, and over the ankle. Press your heel all the way to the top of your foot.

If you feel any pain at any point you have found a spasm in the muscle. STOP and put sustained pressure on the point. Do this several (8-10) times, trying to increase the pressure with each pass.

As you are pressing down onto the muscle, stretch it toward the direction of your foot. As you lengthen the muscle fibers you are relieving the tension from the tendons, you are also drawing fresh blood into the muscle, and you are pressing the fibers back down onto the bone.

Since this can be a tender area, only use enough pressure to work the muscle, but still be tolerable. The chances are that you will not get this muscle to be pain-free after just one treatment, although the pain in the ankle should lessen with the first treatment. Do it for several days in a row.

Immediately next to the tibialis anterior is a muscle called the Extensor Digitorum Longus. This muscle travels down the outside of your leg along with the peroneal muscles. They insert on the top of your foot and on the outside of the foot. Together they lift your foot and angle it so pressure falls onto your big toe. TP Chart 15 demonstrates the pain pattern for the Tibialis Anterior, and for the Extensor Digitorum Longus.

Pain in the ankle can be caused by the peroneal muscles; TP Chart 17 demonstrates that pain pattern.

The way to stretch the tibialis anterior and the peroneal muscles is to point your toes down as far as you can while turning your foot so the toenails, and the length of your toes, are pressing into the ground. Put pressure onto your toes until you feel the stretch of the muscle.

Another way to stretch the muscles is bending by your knees and sitting on your lower leg while your toes are pointed.

The Calf and Achilles Tendonitis

Jerry is a Triathlete. His goal for the last several years has been to compete in an Ironman distance event. He worked towards it for years, and it was finally in sight. Then he developed Achilles Tendonitis. After a year and a half of trying every remedy doctors had suggested, he was barely able to run three miles before the tendonitis would force him to stop. There was no possible way he was going to be able to train enough to compete.

Have your legs ever gotten so tired that they throbbed? Do you get cramps in your calf? Have you been diagnosed as having "Achilles Tendonitis"? Have you ever had a heel spur? Often these are the natural responses of the body to contracted muscle fibers in the calf muscles.

Runners have a propensity to Achilles Tendonitis. This is the condition that occurs when the two muscles of the calf are pulling so tightly onto the tendon that they are actually trying to tear the tendon off the bone!

As the muscles shorten, the tendon pulls, and you lift your heel. However, as the muscle goes into a shortened state, and stays there while you are putting your foot down flat on the ground, the tendon is being pulled so severely that it can either tear away from the bone, rupture the tendon, or cause a heel spur. This last condition, heel spurs, happen because the muscle is trying to tear the tendon from the heel, and the body sends bone cells to hold onto the tendon. This keeps going, the muscle pulling and the body sending bone cells, until a spur developes.

An inflammation at the insertion point of the Achilles tendon is the first step toward potentially tearing the Achilles tendon. Medications may relieve this pain, or may simply take away the inflammatory response, but they only mask the symptoms while ignoring the cause. It is vital to release the spasms in the two calf muscles: the gastrocneimus (gastroc for short) and the soleus!

Heel Striker Pain

Another condition that is often found in athletes is extreme tenderness on the bottom of the heel, and possibly along the inside, and outside, border of the foot. It is possible that the bone is bruised from hitting the ground, with great force, with each step. A bone bruise can take a long time to heal. However, contractions in the gastroc and soleus can also cause pain to radiate through the heel and the foot. The treatment is the same as for Achilles tendonitis. The result may be slower than the Achilles tendonitis treatment, but it will help ease it immediately, and with frequent treatments, the pain will eventually disappear.

As you look at the muscle chart for the gastroc and the soleus, notice how they merge into the tendon. To release the tension on the spasm you will need to treat the calf muscles.

We have noticed that most people have seen, or used, the stretch for the "gastroc" muscle - the top muscle of the calf - but they aren't aware that there are two muscles in the calf. Under the "gastroc" is a muscle that, while hidden from view, is just as important when addressing pain in the calf or heel. That muscle is called the soleus.

Take a look at TP Chart 14 and you can see the trigger points on the gastroc. The soleus is under the gastroc, and can't be clearly shown on these charts. Both of these muscles insert into the Achilles tendon, the thick band at the back of your ankle, and then go to the heel bone. When they contract, your heel is lifted off the floor, and you are standing on your toes. The difficulty arises because even those people who do stretch frequently ignore the soleus, only doing the stretch that works on the "gastroc"

Before going into the treatment for these two muscles, look at TP Chart 13 – piriformis, TP Chart 14, and TP Chart 17 – gluteus minimus. You'll notice that calf pain comes not only from the calf, but from muscles far from the calf, so if local treatment doesn't help, look for the spasm elsewhere.

Prior to treatment, warm the muscles whenever possible. Use a heating pad for 5 minutes, and do some gentle stretching by putting your leg out straight, bring your toes up toward your shinbone, then rotate your foot in a circular direction.

As you move along the muscle during the following treatments, if you find a painful "bump", that is the spasm that needs to be pressed out!

Because they are on top of each other, the treatment will melt spasms in both of the lower leg muscles. Begin very gently with these treatments, calves can be quite painful! If you're flexible it's easy to do these treatments by using your shinbone as a rolling pin, so let's begin by demonstrating how to treat the right leg.

Kneel on the floor, holding onto a wall, or a chair. Use your shinbone to press down onto your calf.

Alternatively, use an 18" length of dowel (or a rolling pin, in a pinch). Start up as close to your knee as you can get, DON'T PUSH

BEHIND YOUR KNEE, and push it all the way down to your ankle. If you find any especially tender spots, stay on them for about one minute, and then continue down to the ankle. Do this several times on both legs.

Because you run on a wide variety of surfaces, and in all kinds of weather, you can't always kneel down. This was brought to our attention while working with Jerry, the Ironman

Triathlete previously mentioned. We needed to figure out a way that could be done in the cold, wet, weather in Washington State. He discovered how to do the treatment by balancing on a tree or road sign! Since Jerry discovered this technique, here he is demonstrating how to do it.

Hold on to a secure object, bend your knees and put your knee directly onto the calf of your sore leg. Hold this for 60 seconds, and deeply slide your knee down toward your ankle.

Do several passes down the calf in order to work the entire calf muscle.

You can also effectively work on your calf muscles while you sit cross-legged in a chair. Simply put your calf directly on top of your knee - press down- and slide from the top of your calf to your ankle.

Finally, you can do this while you are relaxing! Simply put your calf on top of your bent knee and move your top leg to slide the kneecap under the calf muscle. Go from the top of the calf to the ankle.

Even if you are only feeling pain or tightness in one leg, do both legs. You'll be surprised how painful they both can be.

Muscle Cramps

If you experience a sudden cramp, don't try to stretch out the fiber while the contraction is still happening. A muscle contraction will not stop in the middle of the pull; if you stretch it during the cramp you will be pulling it in the opposite direction and then you may tear the muscle fibers. This is one of the reasons that often a person will feel pain in the muscle long after the cramp has ended.

Instead of stretching and pulling on the muscle fibers, hasten the completion of the cramp by assisting the fibers in their contraction, and then stretch the muscle. The two most common places for muscle cramps are in the calf, and in the arch of the foot.

To hasten the end of a cramp in the calf muscle, tightly grip above and below the muscle – just below the knee and just above the ankle – and push your two hands together, shortening the muscle. This will be extremely painful for about 10 seconds – but the time will still be shorter than you normally experience when your leg cramps.

Hold the muscle together for about 15 seconds and then release. Repeat this same movement to help any last fibers to complete the contraction. The pain will be substantially less during the second movement.

Now you can move into the treatments for the calf muscles – the soleus and gastrocneimus shown in this chapter.

The arch of the foot is treated in a similar manner.

Grip your foot around the ball at the base of the toes, and at the heel. Then push the two ends together as much as possible. This treatment is fast, and less painful, because the muscle is so short.

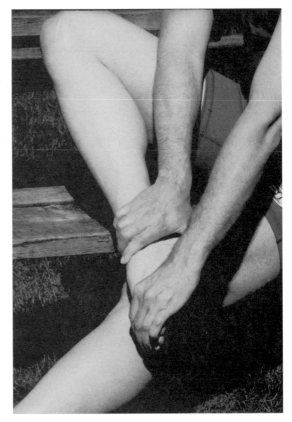

After treating the foot cramp you can proceed to stretch it out by standing up on your toes and leaning forward. You can also push your thumbs deeply along the arch - as if you were trying to lengthen the muscle from the heel toward the toes.

Finally, if your toes begin to cramp, sit down and using your fingers, press deeply in all the areas around the base of the toe, and in the areas in between each of the muscle tendons to the foot. Also, press into the ball of your foot, arch, and work up your leg. There will be places that are very painful – you'll know when you find a spasm. Just hold your finger pressure on it for about 60 seconds; you'll feel it melt away.

Lower Leg Stretches

Most people know about the stretch for the gastroc. We teach it without bending forward to lean on a support, so you can do it any place easily. Look at the pictures as an example of good posture: keeping your back straight will be more comfortable.

To stretch the gastroc, put one leg forward, and the other back. Keeping your foot flat on the floor, bend the forward knee.

To stretch the soleus, stay in the same position as for the gastroc, then move your body back a bit and bend your back knee. You will feel the stretch in a totally different location.

We've had runners who are shocked at how different they feel when they stretch the two muscles, instead of just one. The relief felt is wonderful!

Finally, the last lower leg muscle we will work is the Peroneal muscle group. Three muscles that do a multitude of assisting movements. Their primary purpose is to enable you to lift your foot from a flat position to a position where your little toe and outside of your foot are lifted up from the floor. This movement is called aversion.

Recently, in a very short time span, we had three clients who were having a problem with this muscle. One had twisted her ankle while running on an uneven surface; one had broken her leg several months prior; and the third didn't have anything he could blame it on - he just couldn't put pressure on the outside of his foot. In all three cases the peroneals were to blame.

The twisted ankle caused the peroneals to rapidly overstretch, and then spasm as they returned into place. The broken leg bone (fibula) caused the muscle to suddenly contract fully. The muscle

was stretched back into place as the bone was being set, but the contractions were not relieved, and the shortened muscle put pressure on the ankle. Because of their location, the self-treatment is more difficult to do, but it can be done.

Stand up and put your leg onto a chair, or sit on the floor or bed.

Roll your foot out toward your little toe and turn your leg so you can better reach the muscle. Using the length of dowel, press onto the outside border of your leg, just above the ankle. Lean back and slide the pole up your leg, stopping just below the bone of your knee joint.

If you find an area that is especially tender, that is the spasm. Using the dowel, press on it, try to flatten it, and stretch the fibers. These are forgotten muscles, and are rarely stretched, or flushed out by the majority of massage therapists. Yet, a little treatment goes a long way with the peroneals. Flush them out and your ankle will move easier, any nagging discomfort can be quickly relieved.

CHAPTER 12

Foot Pain

All sports that involve landing hard on the foot, such as: running, tennis, soccer, basketball, and a wide assortment of other sports, can cause foot pain. Even swimming and cycling, sports that wouldn't be thought of as stressing the foot, cause cramping, and pain in the top of the foot.

Your feet are your foundation, when they are in pain you can't continue. We are sure you have already found the best footgear for your sport, and that you do the normal care for nails, arch support, and callous removal. We want to discuss how the muscles can cause pain and cramping – and how you can stop it short.

Many of the treatments for the foot are included in the Chapter 11 - The Lower Leg, because the muscles of the lower leg are responsible for the movement of the foot.

It has been our experience that the majority of people, when they feel pain in their foot, would not think to look at the leg as the source of the problem. However, the large majority of time, this is exactly where the problem is occurring.

Pain on the top of the foot, and pain in the arch, is often caused by the tibialis anterior and peroneal muscles on the front and outside of the lower leg. When you are running, you are contracting the tibialis anterior muscle in order to land on your heels, but you don't follow through with pointing your toes at the end of the step. One way to help relieve shin/ankle/foot pain <u>while you are running</u>, is to complete each step by pointing your toes as you push off.

Cycling keeps your ankle bent for hours, which means the tibialis anterior is held in a contracted state for hours. Eventually the muscle shortens (it's called muscle memory) and pulls on the tendon, causing pain at the top of the foot, as well as along the shinbone.

Heel pain and bone spurs are also frequently caused by tightness in the calf muscles. You will not eliminate these pains until you release the spasms in both the gastrocneimus and soleus muscles of the calf.

Plantar Fasciitis

Plantar Fasciitis means "inflammation of the fascia of the muscles on the sole of the foot". The foot has several important muscles that move the toes into various positions.

To treat the muscles of the arch and the sole of the foot, simply put a golf ball on the floor and roll your foot on it. Press it into the arch of your foot and roll it back and forth (from toes to heel & reverse). Go up into your toes, and along both sides of your foot.

There are two other important areas of the body that commonly refer pain to the arch. The first is the Piriformis muscle. This muscle is located under the back pocket of your pants. The muscle crosses over the sciatic nerve, and when it goes into a spasm, it presses the nerve into the bone (called the Greater Sciatic Notch), causing Sciatica. When the sciatic nerve is impinged, you feel pain in your hip, down the back of your leg, and into your arch. The Piriformis muscle is responsible for turning your foot out, which is a very common problem for runners.

The following picture demonstrates an easy way to stretch the piriformis when you have pain while you are exercising, and are you are unable to lie down:

Stand up with your leg out in front of you, your knee locked, and your foot pulled up.

Keep that position and turn your foot all the way into the midline - so your toes are pointing to the back of the opposite ankle. You will feel the stretch in your hip and buttocks.

This is a very important stretch for anyone who sits a lot, runs, or climbs stairs.

Another important area that causes plantar fasciitis, and Achilles tendonitis, is the muscles of your calf. A spasm here will try to pull the Achilles tendon away from its insertion at the heel, and will refer pain to the arch.

As demonstrated in Chapter 11 – The Lower Leg, the best way (there are several) to treat this is to sit down, cross your legs (sore leg on top) and press the center of your calf muscle directly into the knee of the opposite leg (see treatment in lower leg). Use your locked hands to add pressure on the top leg, pushing it further into the bottom legs kneecap. Make sure your foot/ankle is relaxed. Now, pull your top leg up, so the kneecap slides from the top of the calf down toward the ankle.

This treatment may be painful, especially as it passes over the spasm. Stay well within your tolerance level, this treatment may take several passes before the spasm begins to go down. Turn your top leg to try to treat the entire calf muscle.

Heel Pain (also see Chapter 11 – The Lower Leg)

Pain in the heel of the foot - on the bottom, inside border is also caused by the calf muscles. One would think of it as a "bone spur" in the pad of the heel, but in this case, it isn't. Work the calf muscles with your opposite knee, it is an important treatment when you have heel pain.

After releasing the calf muscles, use your fingers to deeply press down on the insertion point of the Achilles tendon, all the way down to the bottom of the heel. It takes a long time to really work this one out - but every time you do it you will have pain relief for a few hours. Gradually it getts better and better - hurting less and the treatment lasts for a longer time.

Sharp Pain in the Ball of your foot and cramping of the Toes

When this happens you may have spasms in the lumbrical muscles. These are small muscles that go between each of the tarsal bones in your feet, and up to the first joint in your toes. The tarsal bones are the long bones in your feet, that lead up to your toes.

Because of their insertion into other, longer, muscles, the action of the lumbricals is to assist in curling your toes up, and down.

As you are exercising, you are probably holding your toes one way, or the other, for long periods of time. Ultimately the muscles shorten (called muscle memory).

When they shorten, and you try to move your toes in the opposite direction, the muscle pulls on the insertion point. It feels like a sharp pin has been stuck into your foot - in between the toes, but down a bit toward the meaty part of the ball of your foot (base of your toes).

To treat them, take off your shoe. Cross your leg over so you can easily press into the ball of your foot, and also the top of your foot, between the tarsal bones. You'll just have room between the tendons, and the tarsal bones, for one fingertip. Press around, you'll find the spasms. It will feel like a tiny pea, or a tiny pebble.

Press your fingers deeply into your foot, go in between all the tendons, between the bones, wherever you can find a painful point - that is a spasm.

When you find the spasm, hold pressure on it, as deep as is comfortable - and you'll feel it ease up. As it is getting less painful, the muscle spasm is melting. We suggest you keep poking around and look for any other spasms that may have developed in your feet.

A golf ball is a wonderful thing to stand on and roll around under your toes, ball of the foot, arch, and heel. The dowel is another perfect object because it is smooth, it rolls, and it covers the entire bottom of the foot at the same time.

It will help you to find, and treat, many spasms. It's like a quick "foot reflexology" treatment. Your feet will feel great!

CHAPTER 13

Getting Race Ready

At the Start Line...or before your long training run

Congratulations! It's all come together and you are at the Start Line of the race. Your heart is pumping...your mind is rushing from place to place...you're warming up your muscles and trying to keep your thoughts calm by chatting with fellow runners. You only have 10 minutes to go and your body will be pushed to its limit – or beyond!

Take this time to prepare your muscles for the task ahead, focus your thoughts in a direction that will enhance your ability. It is important that you increase the circulation to each muscle group, and to assure that your joints are as flexible as possible. This is the pinnacle of your preparation and training. Use these minutes wisely!

As best as you can under the circumstances, try to find a space away from the hub of the action. If you can sit on the grass it would be ideal. To prepare your muscles and joints you will need just five minutes of concentrated efforts that will bring huge results.

Before you sit down, close your eyes, take in two or three slow deep breaths, visualizing oxygen filling your lungs completely and sending nutrients to each of your muscles. "Feel" a wave of relaxation flow down your body, from your head to your toes. "See" your muscles untying, lining up like elastic bands, well-tuned for the task before them. This 30-second meditation will actually cause your muscles to release tension that has been building as you moved toward the Start line.

- Begin your stretches with your psoas muscle (Page 62), doing the slow back and forth movement at least 5 times.

- Continue by doing one 30-second stretch for both sides of your quadratus lumborum (Page 70)

- Lie down in the grass (or if impossible, lean up against a tree or building) and bring one knee close to your body.

Push it toward the opposite side and hold on to your ankle. Slowly move your lower leg up toward your shoulder and stretch your lateral rotator muscles, especially the piriformis. (Page 77)

- Lean over in a sitting position and placing your flat hands on the ground, slowly straighten your legs to stretch your hamstrings. Don't overdo it, just a nice gentle stretch. (Page 93)

- Sit down on the ground and using your forearm, push down on your quads, moving toward your knee. One or two passes is all that is necessary to flush out any lactic acid and bring in fresh blood (Page 90)

- Bend your knees and use the heel of your hand to push the lactic acid from your tibialis anterior muscle, stretching the fibers toward your ankle (Page 97).

- Gently push your knee down your calf muscles. Prior to a race you don't want to press too deeply onto this muscle. One pass on the inside-middle-outside is enough. This isn't a time to work out spasms so DO NOT be pressing in deeply. Your intention is to lengthen the fibers and draw blood into the muscle to nourish it as you run. (Page 109)

- If possible, find a big rock and step on it, rotating your feet to warm up the muscles of your arch and toes.

- Stand up and slowly rotate your entire body in every direction. Move your shoulders, your hips, your neck, in circular directions. All the while, visualize your muscles as strong, elastic bands.

Finish your 5 minute warm-up with another deep breath. Keep your thoughts on seeing yourself as you cross the finish line.

You are now ready to race – Good Luck!

While You Are Running

Your mind is all over the place. It goes from thinking of nothing, to watching the crowd, to thinking about aches and pains, and wondering if you are going to make it to the end.

It's amazing how the mind controls the physiology of the body, and it's important to focus your attention on what you DO want, keeping your thoughts away from what you DON'T want. If you allow your mind to focus on pain, it will intensify, so you need to be consciously aware when you find your thoughts taking you away from your goal.

When you are aware of pain, first think of what you can do to reverse it while you continue running. There are a few things that can help without causing you to lose time:

- If your shins or the top of your foot/ankle start to hurt, your tibialis anterior muscle is in spasm. You can stretch it while you run by exaggerating the movement of pointing your toes toward the back as you push-off from your step.

- Calf pain or Achilles tendonitis pain is caused by some or all of the muscles in your calf going into spasm. Exaggerate your step as you come down on your heel. This will give a slight stretch to the calf muscles

- Occasionally think to arch your back while you run. This will help to stretch the psoas muscle and will prevent, or alleviate, a whole list of possible pains.

- You are breathing deeply as you run, enhance the experience by visualizing oxygen as tiny pellets of nutrition being forced into your muscles.

- If you do stop for a water break, quickly flush down your quads with either the heel of your hand or with your arm. Use a pressure that feels good, you are trying to push out lactic acid that is building up from the muscle action. You will also be drawing in blood so it will help your recovery tomorrow.

- At the water break you can also wrap your hands around your thighs and quickly flush out your hamstrings, and then slide down to your lower leg and squeeze the lactic acid from the muscles of your calf (use your four fingers) and tibialis anterior (using your thumbs).

After The Race

You know the normal routine: drink lots of fluids, avoid chills, walk around to prevent muscles from tightening. You will heal much faster if you add a few things to your post-race routines

Use arnica gel as a lubricant and flush out your muscles from your hips to the arches of your feet. Simply squeeze &/or press your hands into all of your muscles. You are actually pushing the lactic acid out of the fibers. Your muscles are sore, so be gentle with your pressure, but vigorous in your actions.

Many athletes tell us they have success by taking arnica tablets before and after the race – 3 tablets every 15 minutes for two hours. This gets the arnica into the blood stream to heal the muscles from within.
Gently stretch each of the muscles. It is important to be gentle, your muscles are in an injured state, you need to nurture them.

If there is a massage tent, bring your arnica gel and ask the therapist to flush out your legs while using the gel. Ask them to press out the lateral rotator (hip) muscles and lightly stretch your back. Avoid any deep muscle treatments until two or three days after the race.

Get a good nights sleep – you deserve it!

A Few Other Thoughts

Arnica is a 200+ year old homeopathic remedy for muscle bruises. We have been told by many of the athletes who come into the office how taking three arnica tablets every 15 minutes for two hours prior to the race has greatly improved both the pain felt during the race, and also hastened the healing time after the race.

We recommend that you pack a tube of arnica gel into your waist pack for after the race. Generously rub it on your muscles, and keep rubbing it on frequently after the race.

Before you leave home on the day of the race, review the treatment for muscle cramps (Page ???). Hopefully you won't need it. Since stretching a cramping muscle can tear the fibers causing greater pain that can last for several days, it's important to have this technique in the front of your mind should you suddenly need it.

Finally....

Running is a sport that you can enjoy for your entire life.

Be sure to have your annual check-ups, eat properly, stretch, and get enough rest to compensate for the strain you are putting on your body.

If you treat your body right you will be rewarded with years of "Pain-Free Running".

We wish you the very best as you grow in your sport. Please visit us at our forum on www.julstro.com.

PART IV – GLOSSARIES AND TRIGGER POINT / MUSCLE CHARTS

Appendix A - Glossaries

These glossaries are not meant as a medical dictionary. They are included for the convenience of the reader who has little knowledge about the body. Only those terms that are used in this book are included in the Glossary of Terms, and only the major muscles, and not all muscles discussed in the book are listed in the Glossary of Muscles

The explanations have been purposely written in non-technical language. For a more complete glossary, please check any good anatomy and physiology textbook

Glossary of Terms:

Adhesion: When muscle fibers have an injury, they put out a substance that sticks the adjoining fibers to the injured fiber. This allows the injured fiber the opportunity to rest and heal.

Anterior: Toward the front of the body. (i.e.: your chin is anterior, your spine is posterior).

Arnica gel: A topical homeopathic remedy that heals bruised muscles.

Bone spur: A "bump" on a bone. A tight muscle that is attempting to pull its insertion away from the bone frequently causes a spur. The body sends the bone cells to hold the insertion in place.

Brachial Plexus: A group of nerves that originate in the neck and are responsible for the sensations felt in the arm, hand, and parts of the chest and back.

Breastbone: Common name for the sternum.

Carpal tunnel: Found in the wrist, it is an area that is formed by 8 small bones (carpal bones) as the base, and the flexor retinaculum as the bridge. Nine flexor tendons and the medial nerve pass through this area.

Carpal Tunnel Syndrome (CTS): A condition in which the median nerve is being damaged as it passes through the carpal tunnel.

Cervical Vertebrae: Neck bones.

Clavicle (Collarbone): The long bone located at the very top of the chest, it extends from the breastbone to the shoulder.

Collarbone: Common name for the clavicle.

Contraction (of a muscle): The natural movement of a muscle. When a muscle contracts (shortens), a joint moves.

Extensors: Any muscles that draw a limb away from its natural bend, i.e.; the extensors of hand straighten your fingers when they are bent, and the extensors of the leg straighten a bend of the knee.

Flexors: Any muscles that bend a limb; i.e., the flexors of the hand cause you to make a fist, and the flexors of the leg cause you to bend your knee.

Flexor retinaculum: The bridge of the carpal tunnel, the flexor retinaculum is the origin of several of the thumb muscles.

Frozen shoulder: A condition that is caused when many, or all, of the muscles that move the shoulder blade are contracted. The shoulder is unable to move.

Insertion (of a muscle): The area of a bone where the muscle ends. The muscle pulls this point, causing it to move toward the origination of the muscle, i.e., the hamstrings insert on the lower leg, so when they pull the knee bends.

Isometric exercise: A type of exercise where muscle contractions are done with little movement by the body, and are then held static by the muscle.

Julstro Elbow: A multi-functional tool that was specifically designed to help individuals apply pointed pressure to muscle spasms throughout the body.

Julstro Technique: The name of a system of treatments for muscle pains that are caused by repetitive strain injury.

Lactic acid: A natural by-product of muscle action. The body has the mechanism to flush away lactic acid, if it is given sufficient time before more lactic acid is produced.

Lateral: Toward the outer side of the body (i.e.: the arms are lateral to the rib cage).

Ligament: A strong fibrous material that attaches a bone to a bone.

Origin: The point where a muscle or nerve begins. The insertion of a muscle always moves toward the origin.

Lumbar Vertebrae: Spine bones of the low back.

Medial: Toward the center of your body. (I.e.: your chest bone is medial to your shoulder).

Pain referral: The term that describes the condition in which a spasm, or other injury, occurs on one place and is felt in a different place. The area that feels the pain sensation is the pain referral area.

Posterior: Toward the back of your body. (i.e.: your heel is posterior to your toes)

Repetitive strain injury: (RSI) Any muscle injury that is caused by the repeated contraction of a muscle until it either over-contracts or is torn.

Rotator cuff muscles: A group of muscles that enable the arm to rotate at the shoulder joint.

RSI: The abbreviation for Repetitive Strain Injury.

Scapula: (Shoulder Blade) The triangular shaped bone in the upper back. It is the insertion location for many of the muscles that move the arm. This is the area affected by "frozen shoulder".

Shoulder Blade: The common name for the scapula.

Spasm: Involuntary contraction, without release, of a muscle fiber or a group of muscle fibers.

Sternum: (Breastbone) The flat bone in the chest, directly below the chin.

Stiff Neck: When the head cannot move to a full range of motion without pain.

Temporomandibular joint: (TMJ) The hinge joint of the jaw.

Tendon: A strong fibrous material that is the ending portion of the muscle. The tendon inserts onto a bone. Tendons do not have a blood supply, so they heal very slowly.

Tennis Elbow: Also called "briefcase elbow" and many other terms. This condition is caused by the triceps muscle contracting and pulling on the insertion at the elbow. It also prevents the arm from straightening fully without pain in the elbow area.

Thenar muscles: The group name for the muscles that control the thumb.

Thoracic Vertebrae: Spine bones of the mid back.

Trigger Finger: A condition that causes the finger to lock in place when it is bent.

TMJ: See temporomandibular joint.

Trigger points: The name given to spasms, throughout the body, that cause pain to be referred to a different area.

Ulnar bone: The bone of the arm that is easily felt on the same side as the fourth finger (pinky).

Glossary of Muscles

Muscle: [Common nickname] (Muscle Chart #) General location on body

Abdominals: [Abs] (#7) A group of muscles that span the entire lower portion of your anterior trunk.

Biceps: (#2) A muscle that is found on the front of the upper arm.

Deltoid: (#8) Muscle that forms the round part of the upper arm at the shoulder.

Flexors: (#1) A group of separate muscles that work independently to enable your hand to curl into a fist, your fingers to move separately, and your wrist to bend. The tendons of the muscles go through the carpal tunnel.

Erector Spinae: (#10) A group of muscles that move the spine in all directions.

Extensors: (#3, 4, 5) A group of separate muscles that work independently to straighten your fingers and hand from the flexed position, and will pull your hand back (extend).

Gastrocnemius: (gastroc)(#14) Surface calf muscle that pulls the heel up so you can stand on your toes.

Gluteals: (Glutes) Group name for the muscles of the buttocks.

Gluteus Maximus: (#10) (Gluteals) The powerful extensor of the leg, this muscle turns the leg outward.

Gluteus Medius: (#9) (see Gluteals) Located more on the hip than in the buttocks, this muscle is still considered a gluteal muscle. It raises the leg to the side and turns the leg inward.

Gluteus Minimus: (#14, 17) (see Gluteals) Located more on the hip than in the buttocks, this muscle is still considered a gluteal muscle. It raises the leg to the side and turns the leg inward.

Hamstrings: (#13) Muscles in the back part of your thigh. They bend your knee.

Iliopsoas: See "Psoas".

Infraspinatus: (#3) A deep muscle that is located on the lower 2/3 of the shoulder blade.

Latissimus dorsi: (Lats) (#9) Large surface muscle that forms the lower half of the back.

Levator Scapulae: (Levator Scap) (#10) A muscle that goes from the neck to the top of the shoulder blade. It helps you shrug your shoulders.

Opponens Pollicis: Thumb muscle that draws the thumb in toward the palm of the hand.

Pectoralis Major: (#6) The biggest chest muscle.

Pectoralis Minor: (#9) A deep chest muscle that inserts onto the top of the shoulder blade. It helps you shrug your shoulders.

Psoas: (#8, 16) A deep muscle in the abdominal area. It originates on your lumbar vertebrae and inserts into your thighbone.

Quadriceps: (Quads) (#16) Muscles in the front part of your thigh. The "quads" straighten your leg.

Quadratus Lumborum: (QL) (#11) A low back muscle that bends you to the side.

Rhomboid: (#12) Deep muscle that is between the spinal column and the shoulder blade. This muscle pulls the shoulder blades together.

Scalenes: (#1) Muscles of the neck that bring your head down, as if to say "yes". The nerves of the arm pass through these muscles.

SCM (see Sternocleidomastoid)

Serratus Anterior: (#8) A muscle of the chest that is under your arm.

Soleus: (#14) Deep muscle of the calf that works with the gastrocnemius muscle.

Sternalis: (#6) A chest muscle that will cause pain in the chest bone, across the anterior shoulder and down the arm.

Sternocleidomastoid: (#18) A neck muscle that turns your head in the opposite direction.

Subclavius: (#9) Small muscle located directly under your collarbone, near the center of your body.

Supraspinatus: (#10) A deep muscle that is on the top of the shoulder blade. It helps lift your arm.

Tibialis anterior: (T.B.Ant.) (#15) The primary muscle next to the shinbone, it pulls your foot up to lift your toes off the floor.

Trapezius: (Traps) (#6) A large diamond-shaped surface muscle that forms the upper back and curve of the shoulder.

Triceps: (#3, 4) The muscles that are found on the back of the upper arm.

Table of Trigger Point Charts

Table of Muscle Charts

APPENDIX B

Trigger Point chart #1
Arms and Hands:
Scalenes and Flexors

FLEXOR

FLEXOR

FLEXOR

FLEXOR

SCALENES

LEGEND

⊗ TRIGGER POINT

MODERATE TO HIGH PAIN

LOW TO MODERATE PAIN
OR NUMBNESS

130

Trigger Point chart #2
Shoulder and Arm:
Brachalis, Biceps,
Supinator, Palmaris

LEGEND

⊗ TRIGGER POINT

 MODERATE TO HIGH PAIN

 LOW TO MODERATE PAIN
 OR NUMBNESS

SUPINATOR

BRACHALIS

PALMARIS

BICEPS

ᕗ JULSTRO

Trigger Point chart #3
Shoulder and Arm:
Infraspinatus, Triceps,
Extensor Carpi Ulnaris

LEGEND

⊗ TRIGGER POINT

MODERATE TO HIGH PAIN

LOW TO MODERATE PAIN OR NUMBNESS

Trigger Point chart #4
Arms

LEGEND

⊗ TRIGGER POINT

▬ MODERATE TO HIGH PAIN

▬ LOW TO MODERATE PAIN
OR NUMBNESS

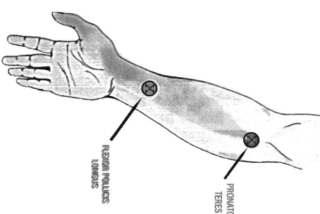

FLEXOR POLLICIS
LONGUS

PRONATOR
TERES

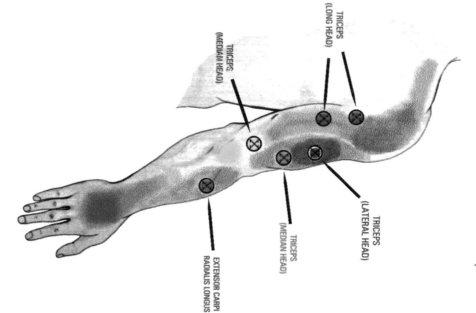

TRICEPS
(LONG HEAD)

TRICEPS
(MEDIAN HEAD)

TRICEPS
(LATERAL HEAD)

TRICEPS
(MEDIAN HEAD)

EXTENSOR CARPI
RADIALIS LONGUS

Trigger Point chart #5
Forearm and Hand

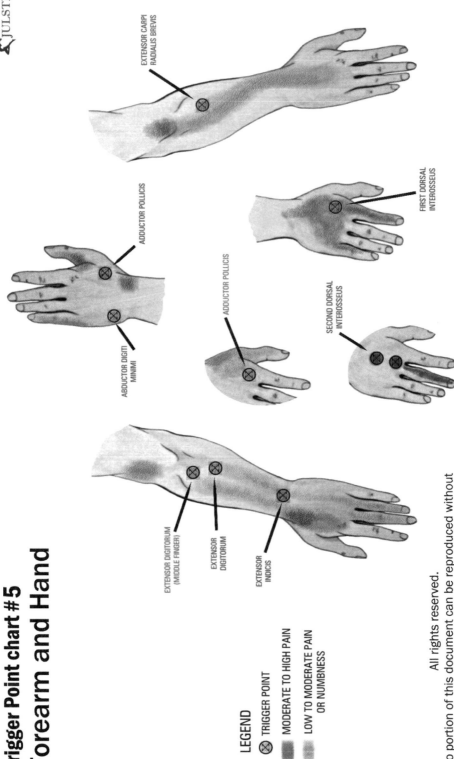

LEGEND

⊗ TRIGGER POINT

MODERATE TO HIGH PAIN

LOW TO MODERATE PAIN OR NUMBNESS

EXTENSOR CARPI RADIALIS BREVIS

ADDUCTOR POLICIS

FIRST DORSAL INTEROSSEUS

ABDUCTOR DIGITI MINIMI

ADDUCTOR POLICIS

SECOND DORSAL INTEROSSEUS

EXTENSOR DIGITORUM (MIDDLE FINGER)

EXTENSOR DIGITORUM

EXTENSOR INDICIS

JULSTRO

134

Trigger Point chart #6
Neck, Shoulder, Chest:
Trapezius, Sternalis, Pectoralis

LEGEND

⊗ TRIGGER POINT

MODERATE TO HIGH PAIN

LOW TO MODERATE PAIN OR NUMBNESS

UPPER TRAPEZIUS

STERNALIS

PECTORALIS MAJOR

🐾 JULSTRO

Trigger Point chart #7
Upper Body:
Pectoralis Major,
External Oblique,
Rectus Abdominus,
McBurney's Point

PECTORALIS MAJOR

EXTERNAL OBLIQUE

EXTERNAL OBLIQUE

RECTUS ABDOMINIS

McBURNEY'S POINT

RECTUS ABDOMINIS

LEGEND

⊗ TRIGGER POINT

MODERATE TO HIGH PAIN

LOW TO MODERATE PAIN OR NUMBNESS

JULSTRO

Trigger Point chart #8
Upper Body:
Serratus Anterior,
Pectroalis,
Anterior Deltoid,
Iliopsoas (Psoas)

LEGEND

⊗ TRIGGER POINT

MODERATE TO HIGH PAIN

LOW TO MODERATE PAIN OR NUMBNESS

SERRATUS ANTERIOR

ILIOPSOAS (DEEP)

ILIOPSOAS

PECTORALIS MAJOR

ANTERIOR DELTOID

⅃ JULSTRO

137

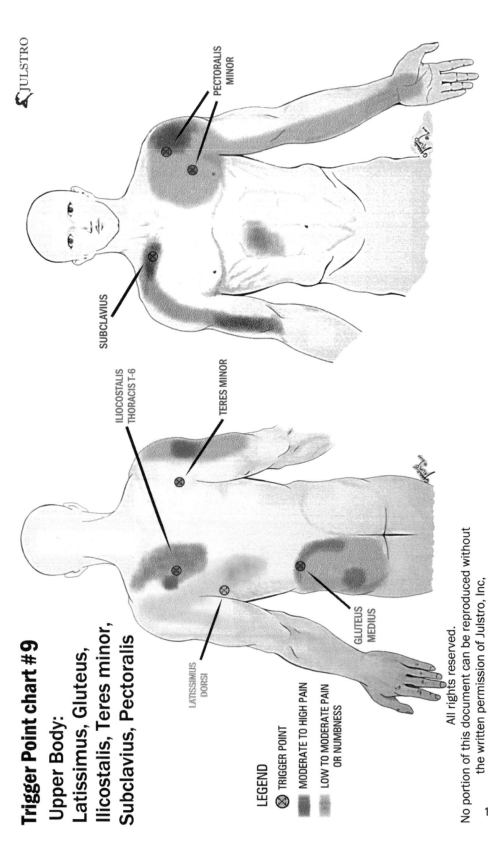

Trigger Point chart #9
Upper Body:
Latissimus, Gluteus, Ilicostalis, Teres minor, Subclavius, Pectoralis

PECTORALIS MINOR

SUBCLAVIUS

ILIOCOSTALIS THORACIS T-6

TERES MINOR

LATISSIMUS DORSI

GLUTEUS MEDIUS

LEGEND
⊗ TRIGGER POINT
MODERATE TO HIGH PAIN
LOW TO MODERATE PAIN OR NUMBNESS

JULSTRO

Trigger Point chart #10
Shoulder, Back
and Neck

LEGEND
⊗ TRIGGER POINT
███ MODERATE TO HIGH PAIN
▓▓▓ LOW TO MODERATE PAIN
OR NUMBNESS

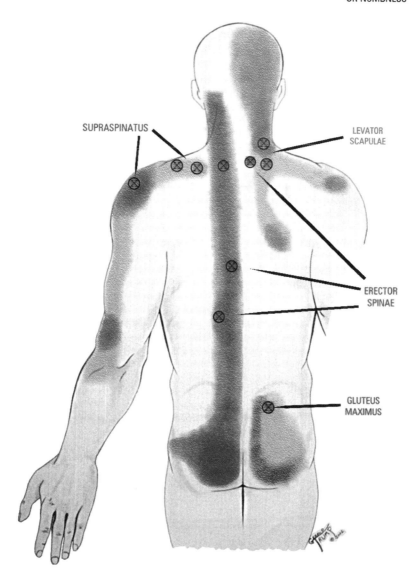

SUPRASPINATUS

LEVATOR
SCAPULAE

ERECTOR
SPINAE

GLUTEUS
MAXIMUS

Trigger Point chart #11
Shoulder and Back:
Trapezius, Deltoid,
Quadratus Lumborum

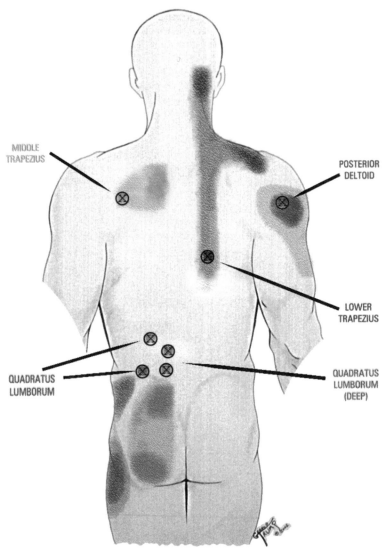

MIDDLE
TRAPEZIUS

POSTERIOR
DELTOID

LOWER
TRAPEZIUS

QUADRATUS
LUMBORUM

QUADRATUS
LUMBORUM
(DEEP)

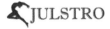

JULSTRO

Trigger Point chart #12
Upper Back:
Iliocostalis,
Rhomboids

ILIOCOSTALIS
THORACIS T-6

RHOMBOIDS

Trigger Point chart #13
Legs, Posterior: Piriformis, Hamstrings

PIRIFORMIS

HAMSTRINGS

⚡JULSTRO

Trigger Point chart #14
Legs, Posterior:

GLUTEUS MINIMUS

BICEPS FEMORIS

GASTROC NEMIUS

SOLEUS

GASTROC

SOLEUS

𝒮JULSTRO

Trigger Point chart #15
Leg, Foot(Anterior)

SARTORIUS

ADDUCTOR
LONGUS

GRACILIS

VASTUS
MEDIALIS

EXTENSOR
DIGITORUM
LONGUS

TIBIALIS
ANTERIOR

ABDUCTOR
HALLUCIS

⟨JULSTRO

Trigger Point chart # 16
Iliopsoas (Psoas), Quadricep

ILIOPSOAS

ILIOPSOAS (DEEP)

SAME POINT

LATERAL QUADRICEP

𝄢 JULSTRO

Trigger Point chart #17
Leg, foot

TENSOR
FASCIAE
LATAE

GLUTEUS
MINIMUS

VASTUS
LATERALIS

PERONEUS
LONGUS

EXTENSOR
DIGITORUM
BREVIS

JULSTRO

Trigger Point chart #18
Head, Neck

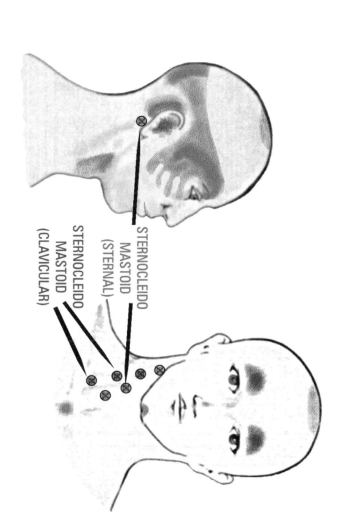

LEGEND

⊗ TRIGGER POINT

MODERATE TO HIGH PAIN

LOW TO MODERATE PAIN
OR NUMBNESS

STERNOCLEIDO
MASTOID
(STERNAL)

STERNOCLEIDO
MASTOID
(CLAVICULAR)

⅃JULSTRO

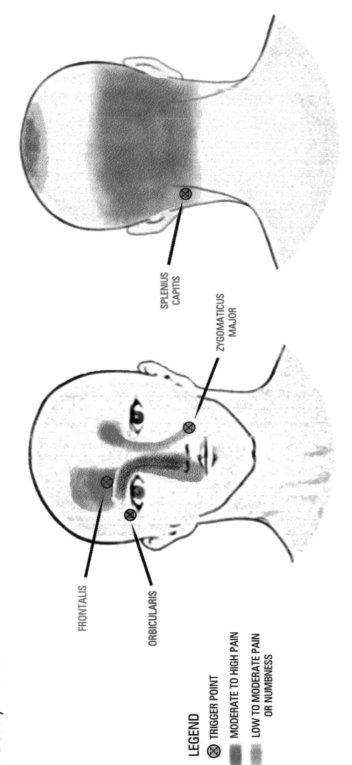

Trigger Point chart #19
Head, Face

ZYGOMATICUS
MAJOR

SPLENIUS
CAPITIS

FRONTALIS

ORBICULARIS

LEGEND

⊗ TRIGGER POINT

MODERATE TO HIGH PAIN

LOW TO MODERATE PAIN
OR NUMBNESS

JULSTRO

Trigger Point chart #20
Head

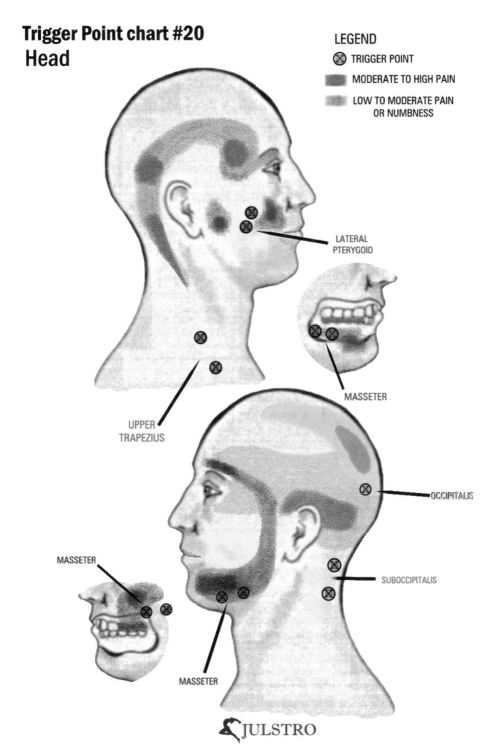

149

Trigger Point chart #21
Face

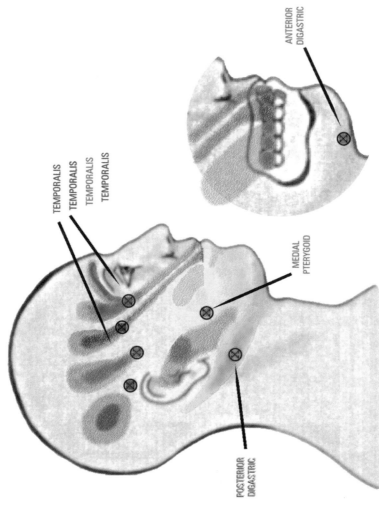

TEMPORALIS
TEMPORALIS
TEMPORALIS
TEMPORALIS

ANTERIOR DIGASTRIC

MEDIAL PTERYGOID

POSTERIOR DIGASTRIC

LEGEND

⊗ TRIGGER POINT

█ MODERATE TO HIGH PAIN

█ LOW TO MODERATE PAIN
   OR NUMBNESS

150

Trigger Point chart #22
Hand

ADDUCTOR
POLLICIS

OPPONENS
POLLICIS

JULSTRO

151

Appendix C – Muscle Charts

This information is provided as a general reference. If you desire the precise sites of Origin & Insertion, and the technical term for the Action of a muscle, look in a good anatomy textbook.

O – Origin, I – Insertion. A – Action.

Muscle chart #1
Arms and Hands:
Scalenes and Flexors

The following information is provided as a general reference. If you desire the precise sites of Origin & Insertion, and the technical term for the Action of a muscle, look in a good anatomy textbook.
O - is Origin. I - is Insertion. A - is Action

JULSTRO

FLEXORS

Just above or below the inside elbow O

| At the wrist, hand &-Or fingers

A - Curls fingers into hand and hand towards underside of forearm

SCALENES

O Cervical Vertebre (C2-7)

| First rib

A-Brings head forward and down

154

Muscle chart #2
Arms and Hands:
Biceps, Supinator,
Brachialis, Palmaris

The following information is provided as a general reference. If you desire
the precise sites of Origin & Insertion, and the technical term for the Action of a muscle,
look in a good anatomy textbook.

O - is Origin. I - is Insertion. A - is Action

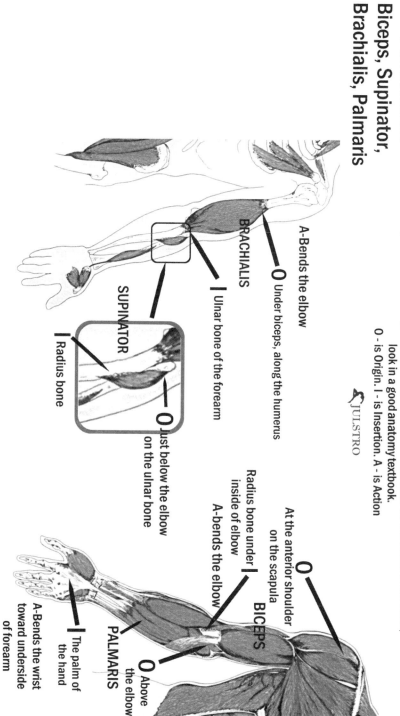

JULSTRO

BRACHIALIS

A-Bends the elbow

O Under biceps, along the humerus

I Ulnar bone of the forearm

SUPINATOR

I Radius bone

O Just below the elbow
on the ulnar bone

At the anterior shoulder
on the scapula

O

Radius bone under
inside of elbow

A-bends the elbow

BICEPS

O Above
the elbow

PALMARIS

I The palm of
the hand

A-Bends the wrist
toward underside
of forearm

155

Muscle chart #3
Arm and Hand:
Infraspinatus,
Triceps,
Extensor Carpi Ulnaris

The following information is provided as a general reference. If you desire the precise sites of Origin & Insertion, and the technical term for the Action of a muscle, look in a good anatomy textbook.

O - is Origin. I - is Insertion. A - is Action

JULSTRO

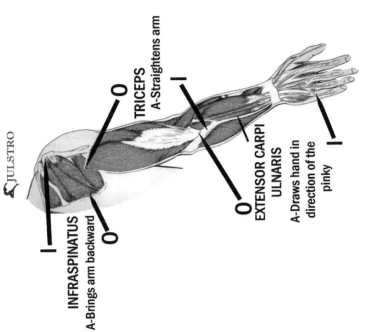

INFRASPINATUS
A-Brings arm backward

TRICEPS
A-Straightens arm

EXTENSOR CARPI ULNARIS
A-Draws hand in direction of the pinky

Muscle chart #4
Arm and Hand:
Flexor, Triceps,
Pronator, Extensor

The following information is provided as a general reference. If you desire
the precise sites of Origin & Insertion, and the technical term for the Action of a muscle,
look in a good anatomy textbook.
O - is Origin. I - is Insertion. A - is Action

🐾 JULSTRO

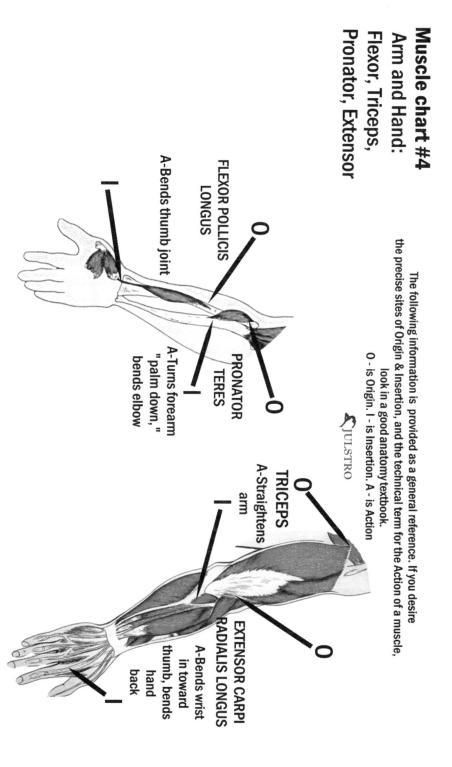

FLEXOR POLLICIS
LONGUS

A-Bends thumb joint

PRONATOR
TERES

A-Turns forearm
"palm down,"
bends elbow

TRICEPS
A-Straightens
arm

EXTENSOR CARPI
RADIALIS LONGUS

A-Bends wrist
in toward
thumb, bends
hand
back

Muscle chart #5
Arm and Hand:
Extensors

The following information is provided as a general reference. If you desire
the precise sites of Origin & Insertion, and the technical term for the Action of a muscle,
look in a good anatomy textbook.
O - is Origin. I - is Insertion. A - is Action

JULSTRO

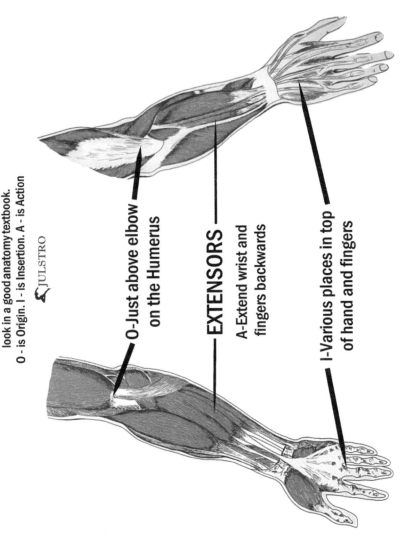

O-Just above elbow
on the Humerus

EXTENSORS

A-Extend wrist and
fingers backwards

I-Various places in top
of hand and fingers

Muscle chart #6
Shoulder, Chest:
Trapezius,
Sternalis,
Pectoralis

The following information is provided as a general reference. If you desire
the precise sites of Origin & Insertion, and the technical term for the Action of a muscle,
look in a good anatomy textbook.
O - is Origin, I - is Insertion, A - is Action

🔥JULSTRO

TRAPEZIUS

A-Moves shoulders up,
down and toward spine

STERNALIS
A-protects the sternum

PECTORALIS
MAJOR

A-Rotates the upper
arm in toward the body

Muscle chart #7
Abdominals

The following information is provided as a general reference. If you desire the precise sites of Origin & Insertion, and the technical term for the Action of a muscle, look in a good anatomy textbook.

O - is Origin. I - is Insertion. A - is Action

🐾 JULSTRO

O
Lower 8 ribs

EXTERNAL OBLIQUES

A-Bends body to the side
I

I
RECTUS ABDOMINUS

A-Bends trunk forward

O

Muscle chart #8

Body:
Serratus, Deltoid,
Iliopsoas (Psoas)

The following information is provided as a general reference. If you desire the precise sites of Origin & Insertion, and the technical term for the Action of a muscle, look in a good anatomy textbook.

O - is Origin. I - is Insertion. A - is Action

↯JULSTRO

SERRATUS
ANTERIOR

A-Draws shoulders
toward the front

ANTERIOR
DELTOID

A-Lifts arm in
front of body,
rotates arm
toward midline

ILIOPSOAS

A-Bends trunk
forward, rotates
thigh away from
the body

161

Muscle chart #9

Shoulder, Hip:
Teres, Latissimus,
Subclavius, Pectoralis,
Gluteus Medius

The following information is provided as a general reference. If you desire
the precise sites of Origin & Insertion, and the technical term for the Action of a muscle,
look in a good anatomy textbook.

O - is Origin. I - is Insertion. A - is Action

JULSTRO

A-Stabilizes collarbone

SUBCLAVIUS O

PECTORALIS
MINOR O

A-Draws shoulder forward
and down

TERES
MINOR

A-Draws arm back
and rotates to the back

GLUTEUS
MEDIUS

A-Lifts leg sideways
away from the body
and rotates leg toward
the midline

LATISSIMUS
DORSI

A-Draws arm down
and rotates in

Muscle chart #10
Shoulder, Back, Hip:

The following information is provided as a general reference. If you desire the precise sites of Origin & Insertion, and the technical term for the Action of a muscle, look in a good anatomy textbook.

O - is Origin. I - is Insertion. A - is Action

JULSTRO

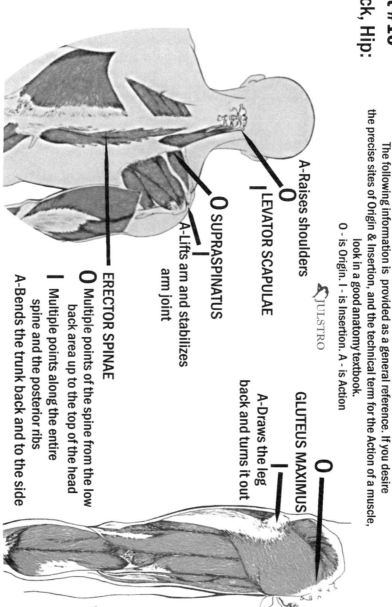

A-Raises shoulders

O

I LEVATOR SCAPULAE

O SUPRASPINATUS

A-Lifts arm and stabilizes arm joint

ERECTOR SPINAE

O Multiple points of the spine from the low back area up to the top of the head

I Multiple points along the entire spine and the posterior ribs

A-Bends the trunk back and to the side

GLUTEUS MAXIMUS

O

I

A-Draws the leg back and turns it out

Muscle chart #11
Low Back:
Quadratus Lumborum

The following information is provided as a general reference. If you desire the precise sites of Origin & Insertion, and the technical term for the Action of a muscle, look in a good anatomy textbook.

O - is Origin. I - is Insertion. A - is Action

JULSTRO

I

QUADRATUS
LUMBORUM

A-Bends body to the
side (or raises the hip)

O

164

Muscle chart #12
Back:
Rhomboids

The following information is provided as a general reference. If you desire
the precise sites of Origin & Insertion, and the technical term for the Action of a muscle,
look in a good anatomy textbook.

O - is Origin. I - is Insertion. A - is Action

𝕁 JULSTRO

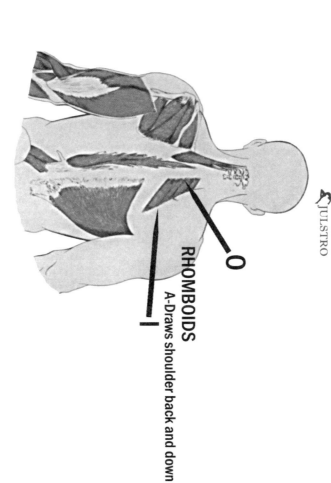

RHOMBOIDS
A-Draws shoulder back and down

O

I

Muscle chart #13
Hamstrings, Piriformis

The following information is provided as a general reference. If you desire the precise sites of Origin & Insertion, and the technical term for the Action of a muscle, look in a good anatomy textbook.

O - is Origin. I - is Insertion. A - is Action

JULSTRO

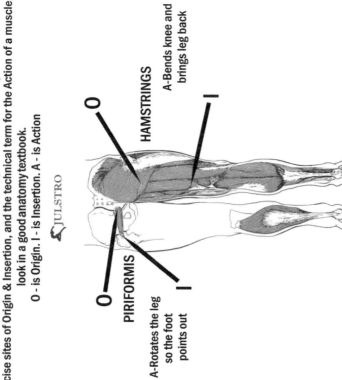

PIRIFORMIS

A-Rotates the leg so the foot points out

HAMSTRINGS

A-Bends knee and brings leg back

Muscle chart #14
Leg:
Gluteus, Soleus, Gastroc

The following information is provided as a general reference. If you desire the precise sites of Origin & Insertion, and the technical term for the Action of a muscle, look in a good anatomy textbook.

O - is Origin. I - is Insertion. A - is Action

JULSTRO

SOLEUS
A-Brings heel up off of ground

GASTROC
A-Brings heel up off of ground

GLUTEUS MINIMUS
A-Raises leg to the side, & rotates leg toward the midline of the body

Muscle chart #15
Leg. Foot

The following information is provided as a general reference. If you desire the precise sites of Origin & Insertion, and the technical term for the Action of a muscle, look in a good anatomy textbook.

O - is Origin. I - is Insertion. A - is Action

JULSTRO

GRACILIS
A-Bends knee and rotates knee toward centerline of body

SATORIUS
A-Brings leg into "crossed leg" squatting position

ABDUCTOR HALLICUS
A-Curls foot by drawing big toe in toward arch

ADDUCTOR LONGUS
A-Bends the knee forward, flexes the hip

EXTENSOR DIGITORUM
A-Pulls up on toes and assists in raising front of foot off the floor

Muscle chart #16

Leg:
Iliopsoas (Psoas), Quadriceps

The following information is provided as a general reference. If you desire the precise sites of Origin & Insertion, and the technical term for the Action of a muscle, look in a good anatomy textbook.

O - is Origin. I - is Insertion. A - is Action

 JULSTRO

A-Bends the body forward, turns leg out

ILIOPSOAS

O

I

LATERAL QUADRICEP

A-Straightens knee, brings thigh up toward body

THREE DEEP QUADS

RECTUS FEMORIS

O

I

169

Muscle chart #17
Leg, Foot:
Gluteus Minimus,
Tensor Fasciae Latae,
Peroneus Longus,
Extensor Digitorum Brevis

The following information is provided as a general reference. If you desire the precise sites of Origin & Insertion, and the technical term for the Action of a muscle, look in a good anatomy textbook.

O - is Origin. I - is Insertion. A - is Action

JULSTRO

O TENSOR FASCIAE LATAE

A-Stabilizes the knee, assists in bending knee

O PERONEUS LONGUS

A-Lifts outside edge of foot off the floor

I A-Lifts toes off the floor

EXTENSOR DIGITORUM BREVIS

O

O GLUTEUS MINIMUS

A-Draws leg away from the body; rotates thigh toward center

Muscle chart #18
Neck

The following information is provided as a general reference. If you desire
the precise sites of Origin & Insertion, and the technical term for the Action of a muscle,
look in a good anatomy textbook.

O - is Origin. I - is Insertion. A - is Action

JULSTRO

A-Turns head on
opposite direction

STERNOCLEIDOMASTOID

I

O

Makai Press
PUBLICATIONS
PO Box 165, Blauvelt, NY 10913
Julstro, Inc. product information
Telephone: (845) 268-2021
Toll free: 1-866- SELF TREAT (1-866-735-3873)
e-mail: orders@julstro.com WEBSITE: www.julstro.com

Products

E-BOOKS

The "Pain-Free" series of e-books are conveniently sent via email to your computer, with links to the full color Trigger Point Charts, and informative Muscle Charts that guides each Julstro self-treatment.

	Price
The Pain-Free Triathlete	$39.95
The Pain-Free Runner	$12.95
The Pain-Free Swimmer	$12.95

BOOKS

The Pain-Free Runner	$19.95
Shipping	$8.50
(add $2.00 for each additional)	

Carpal Tunnel Syndrome:	
What you don't know CAN hurt you	$9.95
Shipping	$7.50
(add $2.00 for each additional)	

The Pain-Free Triathlete	$46.95
Shipping	$10.50
(add $3.00 for each additional)	

VIDEO

The Julstro self-treatment Video System	
For Carpal Tunnel Syndrome	
And hand and wrist pain	$149.95
Shipping	$15.00
(International orders add $15.00)	

ORDER FORM IS ON THE BACK OF THIS PAGE:
Mail to the address above.

ORDER FORM

The Pain-Free Runner e-book **$12.95**   quantity ☐   total ☐

The Pain-Free Swimmer e-book **$12.95**   quantity ☐   total ☐

The Pain-Free Triathlete e-book **$39.95**   quantity ☐   total ☐

The Pain-Free Runner book **$19.95**   quantity ☐   total ☐

The Pain-Free Triathlete book **$46.95**   quantity ☐   total ☐

Carpal Tunnel Syndrome book **$10.95**   quantity ☐   total ☐

Self Treatment Carpal Tunnel
Video System **$149.95**   quantity ☐   total ☐

Add applicable shipping ☐

Sub total ☐

(New York residents add 7.9% sales tax) ☐

Total Order ☐

Payment: Check ☐   Visa ☐   Master Card ☐   Amex ☐

Shipping and billing address: _____

Name (as it appears on the card): _____

Company (or C/O) _____

Address: _____

| City | State | Zip | Country |

Credit Card number:_____

Expiration Date: _____
Month / Year

Signature: _____

174